Praise for *Praying for Emily*

"Playing in the NFL, I have seen my share of tough individuals who were successful because their opponents were unwilling to match their desire to win. Emily's battle with cancer showed this exact toughness. She would not give up!...The story of Emily overcoming all odds to beat cancer, the most ferocious opponent, is inspiring and reinforces the power of hope."

—Jon Condo, retired All-Pro NFL long snapper

"A truly remarkable and uplifting story that is a page-turner and roller coaster ride of emotion all in one! You won't be able to put it down, and you'll be thrilled that you didn't when you get to the triumphant ending."

—Pamela Oas Williams, film and television producer

"*Praying for Emily* is a thought-provoking and heartfelt account of what it means to face the impossible with prayer. Tom and Kari looked into the eyes of their sick child and did the one thing that cancer (and most of the world) did not expect them to do, believe. Because of their faith, the Whiteheads were not only able to save their child, but in sharing their personal experience and story of unrelenting hope, will save so many more. I believe, and you will, too."

—Lori Rothschild Ansaldi, documentary filmmaker, friend, advocate of life

"This remarkable story is a hero's journey, but it's so much more than that: it is the essence of the power of love. I don't know the meaning of life, but this is pretty darn close!"

—Jason Flom, founder, Lava Media, LLC

Praying for

EMILY

Praying for EMILY

THE FAITH, SCIENCE, and MIRACLES That SAVED OUR DAUGHTER

————— ••●•• —————

TOM, KARI, *and* **EMILY WHITEHEAD**
with **DANELLE MORTON**

FOREWORD BY KEN BURNS

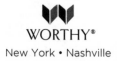

WORTHY®

New York • Nashville

Worthy
Hachette Book Group
1290 Avenue of the Americas, New York, NY 10104
worthypublishing.com
twitter.com/worthypub

First edition: October 2020

Worthy is a division of Hachette Book Group, Inc. The Worthy name and logo are trademarks of Hachette Book Group, Inc.

The publisher is not responsible for websites (or their content) that are not owned by the publisher.

The Hachette Speakers Bureau provides a wide range of authors for speaking events. To find out more, go to www.hachettespeakersbureau.com or call (866) 376-6591.

Library of Congress Control Number: 2020938836

ISBNs: 978-1-5460-3411-7 (hardcover), 978-1-5460-3412-4 (ebook)

Printed in the United States of America

LSC-C

2 2020

*My dad taught me to have **faith**.*
*My mom taught me the importance of **science**.*
*Together we created my **miracle**.*
This is our story.

—Emily Whitehead

CONTENTS

––––––•◦●◦•––––––

FOREWORD

———··•••·———

I meet a lot of everyday heroes in my work: the intrepid explorers who followed Meriwether Lewis and William Clark into the uncharted territories of the Pacific Northwest. The soldiers who lived through the traumatic blood, sweat, and tears of World War II and Vietnam. The athletes who persevered in the face of insidious assaults on their character—and their person—to integrate professional sports.

But none of them is any more heroic than Emily Whitehead, who endured a degree of pain that most of us can barely imagine to prove that a risky, experimental cancer treatment could save her life and the lives of thousands of other children.

She, too, is a pioneer. She, too, is a warrior. She, too, has persevered. As have her parents. As did the thousands of strangers who hoped and prayed for her, united by the simple hashtag #WeBelieve.

We know about the trials and tribulations of scientists and doctors who labor for decades to make revolutionary discoveries, but rarely do we hear about their patients, who are truly on the front lines.

At a time when it seems we can't agree on anything in this culture, we can agree that Emily Whitehead is a hero.

When we first met her, Emily was a five-year-old who spent much of her life in hospitals, surrounded by technology, or at home, trying to live a normal life, as her body began to betray her.

We watched (and filmed) as she hovered near death while doctors feverishly tried to save her. We heaved our own sighs of relief when she went into remission after becoming the first child whose immune cells were successfully trained to fight cancer.

To be honest, we had feared her story would have a far different ending.

Today Emily is a healthy fifteen-year-old who gets straight As, loves art, and, as you are about to see, is able to write about her parents as wisely as they write about her.

Like many teenagers, Emily cares deeply about the challenges her generation faces, from the traumatic effects of bullying to global warming, and she travels the country telling her own story because she believes passionately in doing what she can to raise money for research that will treat other cancers, and save other children (although she also does admit it's "kind of cool" to have your name on T-shirts).

While her parents say she likes being different, even "a little weird because it keeps things interesting," it's also clear (and I hope she doesn't mind my saying it) that the most wonderful thing about her is, simply, that she's a normal teenager—although as the father of one, I know that there is no such thing as a "normal" teenager!

We were fortunate and honored to have had the opportunity to chronicle Emily's journey in our film *Cancer: The Emperor of All Maladies*. I'm so glad her father, her mother, and Emily herself have now given us a chance to hear the rest of her story.

We have a lot to learn from her.

—*Ken Burns*

Chapter 1

ONLY THE STRONGEST CHILDREN ARE PICKED TO FIGHT CANCER

"OK." That was all I could say to the doctor. I briefly glanced back at my mom who was with me in the ER. The doctor went right into the lab values, what was high, what was low, what the normal ranges were, which I didn't hear a word of. I was just thinking, "How am I going to tell Emily? She's only five. She's not going to understand."

—Kari's journal
May 29, 2010

The Friday before Memorial Day, I was up in the bucket truck overlooking a farm field in Grassflat, Pennsylvania, with a crew of linemen replacing cross arms on power poles. We'd met up near dawn among the cornstalks, where we put on big rubber gloves, testing for stray voltage and grounding the lines, before we switched out the cross arms. Getting the job going required all our attention, but as I wrapped the copper tie wire around the insulators on the new arms—something I'd done a thousand times before—I started to pray. At that moment, my wife, Kari, and her mom were with our daughter at the pediatrician, waiting to find out if something was wrong with Emily.

All my thoughts had been about Emily from the moment I'd left home that morning, starting with my memory of the first time I held her in my arms and believed that my little girl could do something that would change the world. I sensed her strong heart and, even as a baby, I saw her joy, and in her eyes that spark of mischief. When Kari and I married in 2001 we struggled at first to start a family. Emily came along in 2005. We had expected Emily would be like Kari: thoughtful, observant, and shy, lover of Disney princesses and the pink and frilly parts of girlhood. I wanted to be the best dad I could be to her, to give her every opportunity, and to protect her. Yet I wasn't sure how to be a good dad to a daughter, having been raised as I was, with two brothers. Right from the start, Emily was her own person: bright, funny, and with a lot to say, even as a toddler.

Like me, she loved the outdoors and had an easy way with people. She was a daddy's girl who laughed at all my jokes, the dumber the better, and, like her dad, she was a prankster. When she heard my car pull in to the driveway, she'd scurry to hide, ready to jump out of a closet or from behind the sofa to startle me or douse me with a squirt gun. Even errands were fun when she was a passenger, strapped into her safety seat, explaining the world to me. She was tender and loving, too, though. When I had to have surgery for my Crohn's disease, she was just three. She decided to sleep on the steps next to the room where I was recovering so she could be there if I needed anything, and she pledged she would grow up to be a doctor so that she could be the one who fixed her daddy.

Emily also inherited her mother's grace and beauty. Often when I got home, I'd find them doing crafts at the kitchen table or curled up in Kari's favorite chair, books stacked on the armrest, because Emily, like Kari, always wanted to read more. Kari and I agreed that we had been blessed with a child who was a perfect balance of the best of Kari and me, and that our family was complete.

As these memories of my beloved little girl flitted through my mind, I tried to stay positive and hope for the best, but all that time something was whispering to me that the news from the doctor was not going to be good.

Two nights before, when Kari got home from work, her mom, Pam—who took care of Emily during the day—said she'd noticed lots of bruises on Emily's arms and legs. Pam said the bruises on Emily's arms could be from the Nerf sword battle she had had with her cousins that afternoon, and the large one on her shin probably was from the stumble she took on our flagstone steps. Emily was strong and full of energy, so we were used to seeing scrapes and bruises on our little girl who was so eager to take on the world. But as Kari dried Emily after her bath that night, she saw more bruises than her mom had seen. Kari counted twenty-one.

Earlier in the week, Kari asked me if I'd noticed that Emily's gums were bleeding when she brushed her teeth. Then Kari remembered that recently Emily had had several nosebleeds. She searched the internet to find a reason for these symptoms. When the online search results highlighted leukemia, Kari didn't think much of it because, other than the bruises, Emily was healthy. She texted her sister Brenda, a nurse, who immediately said these were signs of leukemia. Kari became alarmed. That evening on my way home from work, Brenda called me in tears, saying we had to get Emily to the doctor right away so she could get checked for leukemia.

As I opened my car door in the driveway, I heard Emily's laugh, high and light above the western Pennsylvania birdsong. I followed that sound to the backyard, where I saw her pumping her strong legs on the swing set I'd built for her there. When Emily had said she wanted a swing set, I'd looked in all the big hardware stores but I hadn't found any that seemed strong enough. I wanted a swing that could hold me. That was how I'd know it would be safe enough for her. Finally, I decided to make it myself. When our crews at the electric company switch out the cross arms, we don't throw them away but toss them in a discard pile so the linemen can use them for home projects or contribute them to the community. I picked through that discard pile to find the strongest cross arms to serve as the beams, and sank the swing set's four corners into concrete. Emily came with me to the hardware store to pick out green swing seats and the chain to hold them. I loved watching her swing in them, swooping so high up in the air that I had to reach to give her a push.

When Emily saw me walking toward her, she kicked a flip-flop off the tip of her toe and it smacked me on the shoulder. I staggered around, mortally wounded, a man felled by the weight of her flip-flop. Emily was giggling and I was grinning, but my eyes were on Kari. Her posture was withdrawn, closed in on herself. She was as worried as I was.

"Daddy! Push me!" Emily yelled.

"As soon as I talk with your mom," I said. Kari's eyes met mine when we hugged, and I could see the worry there.

"Look at her," she said. "Is there anything about her that makes you think she's sick?"

"No, except those bruises," I said. "She's rowdy and she plays hard. That's not a sickness."

"I know, and I feel silly rushing her to the doctor," she said. "Dr. Sortor-Thompson is going to think I'm a worrywart."

"I hear you," I said. "But you know what Brenda said."

"I do," Kari said. "I'll call the doctor in the morning."

———•••◆••———

That night I couldn't get to sleep, and Kari was restless. At about one in the morning, Emily came to my side of the bed in tears.

"Daddy!" she whispered. "My knees hurt really bad."

She showed me a tender spot on her knee. I pulled her into the middle of the bed, snug between us. "Just stay here with us," I said.

But as her pain got worse, Kari went to get pain medicine. I rubbed Emily's legs. The combination of the pain medicine and the massage relaxed Emily, who drifted off to sleep. Having her between us soothed us, too. Kari and I fell asleep, the whole family together. I had set my alarm for 4:00 a.m. because I had to go in early for that job in the farm field. But before the alarm sounded, Emily tugged me awake.

"Daddy! Daddy! There's something wrong with my legs!"

I tried to think how to help. "When my joints hurt, nothing feels better than a warm bath," I said.

Kari drew the bath. I carried Emily to the bathroom, trying to have as little contact as possible with her sensitive legs. In the light of the bathroom, I saw bruises on her belly and in the fleshy parts of her underarms—places you don't normally get them. As I lowered her to the water, I noticed reddish-purple dots on her legs. When the back of her legs touched the bathwater, she writhed.

"Owww!" She shrieked. "Get me out! Get me out!"

I wrapped her in a towel and laid her back in our bed to snuggle with

Kari just as my alarm sounded. The last thing I wanted to do was leave them.

———•••●••———

I couldn't stop thinking about them as I rose up in the bucket, watching the sun rise over the field. When I am forty-five feet high above a farm field, I get a view that others pay to see, like the glimpse from the top of a roller-coaster. When the sun pours through the trees, it's like the light in a cathedral, and during those moments I pray. I come from a devout Catholic family, and I go to church when I can, but it is in nature that I sense the presence of God. That morning, I took in a long breath of the sweet, late spring air to try to calm my fears as I cast my eyes beyond the horizon.

My family has lived in Pennsylvania for so long that no one is really sure when the first one of us settled in the western foothills of the Allegheny Mountains, midway between Lake Erie and the Chesapeake Bay. My hometown, Philipsburg, has about 2,700 people, and many of them are related to me. The hills are thick with hardwood trees, maple and birch, and crisscrossed by streams and creeks. As kids, my brothers Jim and Greg and I chased each other through the huckleberry, teaberry, and mountain laurel. We caught frogs and snakes in the pools made by the spring water and floated in the "crick" with our friends in inner tubes, dodging the heat of the summer.

My father was a lineman for the electric company. Eventually all three brothers joined our father on the power lines and, soon after, we started families of our own. One of the many things I loved about my wife, Kari, was that she grew up with three sisters in Woodland, a nearby town even smaller than Philipsburg. When we married, we hoped we would be blessed with a baby. We agreed that the childhood we would offer her would have a strong foundation: safe and secure in a big family, yet in all other ways unbounded. No clock or compass, and with enough free space for any adventure she could dream.

Emily had just turned five. Our families had celebrated her birthday and her graduation from preschool with a big party in our backyard just a few weeks before, and now the summer stretched out ahead of us. She and her half dozen cousins would spend the days swimming, having picnics and Sunday family barbecues in the long afternoons, and fishing at our family camp, until she started kindergarten in the fall. There was no part of our plans that included Emily getting sick.

Up in the bucket looking east, I prayed over and over, like a chant. "Dear Lord, please let Emily be okay. Dear Lord, please." I had shut my eyes to focus on the prayer when my phone vibrated in my back pocket. I yanked off my gloves and swung the bucket away from the wires to take the call safely. The moment I heard Kari's voice, I knew those whispers that something was wrong with Emily had been right.

"You have to come right away," Kari said. "The doctor wants us to go to the emergency room at Clearfield Hospital for blood work. She suspects leukemia."

"I'll leave now," I said. "I'll get there as soon as I can."

It seemed like it took forever to get down from the pole, lift the outriggers that stabilized the truck, and drive out of the field. As the truck rumbled slowly down the dirt road toward State Route 53, my heart ached for Emily. If she had leukemia, nothing would ever be the same for us, or for our families. Our world would go out of balance. I needed to talk to my mom, a retired nurse, so I could hear her tell me things were going to be okay. I tried to punch her number on my phone, but my hands were shaking. I have a tremor in my hand that gets worse when I am under stress, but I kept trying to dial her number as I drove. I wanted to be the one to tell her. I didn't want her to hear this through the family grapevine.

I got the truck back to the shop, headed home to change my clothes, and jumped into my SUV. On the way to the hospital, I stopped by my brother Greg's house, just a few blocks away, to see if our parents were there. Maybe one of them could go with me to the hospital. When I pulled up at Greg's, I was surprised to see Jim, who was supposed to be at work soon. He had stopped in to let Greg's dog out. Jim wasted no time sizing up my state of mind.

"What the hell is wrong with you?" he said as he leaned down to get a good look at me when I rolled down the window.

"Emily's sick. She's got bruises all over. The doctors think it might be leukemia," I said.

"Aw, c'mon! Emily?" Jim said, his big voice booming as he threw his hands up in the air in exasperation. "I've never seen a healthier kid in my life. It's probably nothing. You and Kari worry too much."

"I hope you're right," I said. I kept looking around. "Have you seen Mom and Dad? Where's Greg? Maybe he could come with me."

"I don't know where anyone is," Jim said.

"Well, I can't wait for them," I said, rolling up my window. I needed to hurry.

"It's not going to be anything serious!" Jim shouted after me as I drove away. "Don't drive too fast."

I sped away, and hadn't gotten more than a few blocks before my phone rang. It was Kari.

"It's leukemia," she said softly. "You have to get here. You need to be on the Life Flight, and the doctors want us to choose a hospital."

I took in a big gasp of air.

"Okay," I said, trying to stay calm. "We are going to deal with this. We'll get through it."

When I hung up I felt my chest tighten with fear. I started hyperventilating. I didn't think I could drive to the hospital on my own. And then, at the stoplight downtown, I saw Greg coming the other way in a bucket truck. I called him.

"Pick up, Greg, pick up!" My call went straight to voice mail. I dropped the phone in my lap and started to cry. The cars behind me honked. I don't know how long I'd been stopped at that intersection, but they did.

When I finally got on the freeway, I just floored it.

How will we handle this? I was going to have to be a different kind of father and husband in the months ahead. I would need to keep our family strong so we could fight this together. How would I do that? For now, I just needed to get to Kari and Emily.

Kari called again.

"The blood work shows that Emily's blood cells are ninety percent leukemia cells," Kari said.

"Ninety percent!" I repeated, in shock.

"Her platelets are really low," she said. I heard the beeping sounds of the heart rate monitor and the IV alarm going off in the background. "She has no immune system right now. They gave her an injection of morphine for the pain. The nurses and the doctors are all wearing masks to protect her from germs. They said we need to take her to a children's hospital to see a pediatric oncologist."

"Do they want to Life Flight her because her life is in danger?"

Kari started to sob.

"Kari, Kari," I said. "She cannot see fear in our eyes. She must believe that she can get better. We have to pull it together for Emily."

The staff gave us a choice of two hospitals that could treat Emily's leukemia, Geisinger Medical Center near Danville, Pennsylvania, or Hershey Medical Center. We decided on Hershey, which is affiliated with Kari's alma mater, Penn State, after we called my aunt Laurie, who was in medical school there. She praised the pediatric oncology unit at Hershey, and her endorsement meant a lot to us in the middle of this crisis. Also, Emily was stable by then, so we could drive there without having to take a Life Flight. Aunt Laurie promised to meet us at the entrance.

I walked into the Clearfield ER waiting room and saw Pam and Kari's dad, Robin. Pam had come with Kari and Emily to the pediatrician that morning and I was so grateful Kari had her for company. Pam is petite and reserved, like Kari, with a heartfelt pragmatism. Kari later told me that when the doctor said that Emily had leukemia, she turned to look at her mom and took strength from how calm and steady Pam seemed, taking in everything the doctor said and letting it settle before she expressed an opinion. Kari said she didn't break down until her dad arrived. Kari had fallen into Robin's arms and let him support her. I thanked Robin for being there when I could not, and then I entered the hospital room where Emily and Kari were waiting for me.

I was surprised to see Emily smiling. The morphine took away her pain but had not dulled her spirit. Emily sat like a princess on her throne, propped up by many pillows, watching cartoons and drinking ginger ale, her favorite. When I smiled at Emily, Kari broke into a small smile, too.

I sat at Emily's bedside and took her arm.

"I know you're in a lot of pain and all of this is very scary," I said.

"I'm not in pain right now!" she said, smiling.

"Good, good," I said. "Your mom and I are going to take you to a different hospital because some of the cells in your body aren't working right. That's why your legs hurt so much."

"Daddy, I want you to promise you'll tell me if it's going to hurt," she said.

"We will. If we know it's going to hurt, we'll tell you for sure." I said.

"That's good," Emily said. "Are you and Mommy going to stay with me?"

"We are," I said. "We'll be with you at the hospital to make sure that the doctors get you better fast."

Emily put her little hand over mine and leaned into me. I put my arm around her waist tenderly, remembering all those bruises, and searched my mind for what I could say that would soothe her. I know about being very sick. My Crohn's disease, an inflammatory bowel disease, was diagnosed in my twenties, and the stomach cramps, joint pains, and lack of appetite nearly killed me. I learned that a positive attitude can help. How could I get her to feel that way?

"You know, only the strongest children in the world are picked to fight cancer," I told her, "And you're going to beat it, no matter what."

I had said the wrong thing. Suddenly Emily looked confused and scared, like she was about to cry. No one had said the word *cancer* to her before it came out of my mouth. She was fighting her tears just as I was fighting mine. I had thought I was the one who needed to be strong for Emily, but I recognized then that I had it wrong. Sometimes Emily needed to be strong for me. I drew her a little tighter to me.

"Being afraid doesn't mean that you are not brave," I said. I was stroking her hair slowly, using that rhythm as my anchor to the world, and my tears receded. "We will all cry. We can all cry together."

The nurse came in to check Emily one last time before we put her in the car for the drive to Hershey. Before we got on the road, we swung by the house to pick up a few things and to take Pam back to her car.

When I had finally talked with my mom that afternoon, she'd volunteered to go to our house to pack up what she thought we'd need in Hershey. We had no idea how long we'd be at the hospital. I think of my mom as an angel on earth, someone so generous and openhearted that it's hard to find a moment when she's not doing something for others. Her way of handling pain and fear is to stay busy helping out. When we got to the house, we found that Mom had packed a duffel bag for each of us, a few bags of snacks, a box with some of Emily's one hundred stuffed animals, and a bag filled with books and crafts. I loaded the duffels in the car, but something told me to toss in my hunting binoculars. I had no idea how I'd use them in a hospital, but I grabbed them anyway. Then, just before we got in the car, I told Kari to hold on a second because I wanted to get something else. I ran upstairs to our bedroom and opened the drawer where I kept the Saint Christopher medal my grandmother gave me when I'd gotten sick: an oval of silver on a thick chain. It is a pure silver casting of Saint Christopher with the child up on his shoulder, the one he carries over troubled waters, and the words "St. Christopher Protect Us" etched in the oval that surrounds the saint. I wore it all the time when I was looking for a doctor to cure me. When my grandmother and I prayed for my Crohn's disease to heal, I always held it between my thumb and my forefinger. I wanted to have a link to my grandmother's prayers for my health, which had worked. We needed the same for Emily. I tucked Saint Christopher in my pocket, and then we got going while Emily dozed in the back of our SUV.

Kari and I didn't talk much during the drive. Kari was drained. I wondered what she was thinking, but I couldn't ask because my own mind was so full of worries. How could we do this? What were we going to do about work? How could we support ourselves? I couldn't think about the money. This was going to cost so much more than I could ever imagine. But it didn't matter. We would do whatever it took to have Emily survive. They could take every material possession I had—the house, and the job, everything—as long as they saved Emily. Our families would help us. Our community, too.

Then I looked at Kari. I worried this was going to be more than she could handle, because Emily was everything to her. I could not lose my daughter, or I might lose my wife, too. *Pull it together, now,* I lectured myself. *Be their rock.*

Kari and I would have many decisions to make, and I hoped we would agree on the best course for Emily. Kari is a scientist, a dietitian with a master's degree in nutrition, who is comfortable in the data, the facts. For me, science holds the cure, but it was not everything. In my battle with Crohn's disease, sometimes I have had to defy my doctors. One doctor close to home predicted I would die young because my case was so severe. But when I held the Saint Christopher medal between my fingers, I sensed something—something whispered to me. I somehow knew that there was a specialist out there somewhere who didn't feel the same way this doctor did. I searched until I found a specialist with a treatment and a surgery that saved my life. Science saved me. But I wouldn't have found that solution without listening to those whispers.

Ever since I got sick, my decisions have been guided by these whispers. The word *whisper* isn't exactly right because the whispers don't come in words. I get a sense of something I can't name, a recognition, like a distant voice sounding deep inside. And sometimes I get flashes from the future of things that later come to pass. To hear these, to name them, I have to concentrate as hard as if I'm listening for a whisper.

I would have to stay alert to hear those whispers now that Emily's life hung in the balance. When I am trying to make a big decision, the whispers are hard to hear. I feel them more strongly than other people I know, yet I doubt them just as much. I'd ignored them the night before, when Kari and I assured each other there was nothing wrong with Emily. Kari and I had tried convincing ourselves that Emily was fine. When her gums were bleeding, I'd told her to ease up on the toothbrush. We'd thought the nosebleed the week before was from roughhousing. And the knee pain was just growing pains. But these were all signs of leukemia. If I'd listened to the whispers sooner, would things have been different? I looked at Emily, asleep in the backseat. Her skin was so pale and there were dark circles under her eyes. I hadn't wanted to see these things when I was arguing myself out of believing Emily was sick. This reflex to negate the news we did not want to hear did not serve Emily. I had to concentrate on hearing those whispers, and to consider them wisely, or we would lose Emily.

When I was trying to find a doctor to treat my Crohn's disease, the specialist I found was at Johns Hopkins in Baltimore. The day I went there to have a section of my colon removed, my parents came with me. I was twenty-eight years old, and I had been sick for years. I am six feet five, but I weighed only 168 pounds. In the elevator, I saw a little boy who looked to be about seven or eight years old, in jeans and a T-shirt, bald as bald could be. He had a big grin on his face and was standing at the elevator buttons.

"Hey! How are you doing?" I asked him.

"I'm doing good," he said.

"Are you running the elevator?" I asked.

"I am now," he said. "What floor do you want?"

I asked for the basement and, as the door shut, I couldn't take my eyes off the little boy. His skin was the pale yellow people sometimes get after many rounds of chemotherapy. Why was he in the elevator alone? I guess he sensed my curiosity.

"I'm going to die in six months," he said. "They're doing some tests on me. Maybe what they find might help somebody in the future,"

The elevator door opened, and he flashed us a smile.

"I hope your tests come out okay," he said to us. I waved to him as we exited to find the lab.

If my mom hadn't been standing by my side, I might think I had imagined that boy. He was so calm and cheerful in the face of death that he seemed like someone I had conjured to help me with my own fears.

My Crohn's improved after the surgery, but I thought about him every time I stepped into an elevator. He seemed to be a sign of something that I couldn't see clearly yet. From that day on, whenever I started feeling sorry for myself, or Kari and I faced a big challenge, I'd think of that little boy. "We don't have problems," I'd say. "We can take anything life throws at us. We don't have a child with cancer. Parents who have a child with cancer, now they have real problems."

Now here we were, years later, about to find out what that little boy in the elevator was meant to tell me.

------- ··•·· -------

When we pulled up to the hospital entrance, we were happy to see Aunt Laurie waiting outside on a bench, holding a stuffed animal for Emily. Laurie has thick, curly brown hair and a genial and welcoming smile, but that day we saw the concern on her face. Aunt Laurie is my mom's baby sister, the youngest of nine, and only two years older than I am, so we've always been more like cousins than aunt and nephew. When her husband was killed in a car accident, their children were quite young. She knew she would have to support her family, and she took the bold step of applying to medical school. This year she was in her residency at Hershey. We were so relieved that she would be there for support.

She escorted us through the hospital lobby to the elevators that took us to the seventh floor. The double automatic doors into the pediatric oncology unit made a soft swooshing noise as they opened, the portal to unknown territory. We looked down a long, straight hallway with nine rooms on the left and six on the right, plus a nurses' station. A nurse led us to the first room on the right, apologizing for giving us the smallest room, but, she said, it was the only room available. The room gave me a sense of dread, like something awful was about to happen there. I wondered about the children who had been in that room before Emily.

The nurse who came to check Emily's vitals and take her medical history advised us that we'd have to wait until Tuesday to know what type of leukemia she had because most of the staff was off for the Memorial Day weekend. All they would do for the next three days was keep Emily comfortable with morphine and anti-nausea medicine.

After all the rushing we had just done to get her to Hershey, all our energy now had no place to go. How quickly the world you've built around you retreats when your child gets cancer. Our family shifted from our little house with the big yard and wide-open sky to a cramped room where Emily was kept alive by tubes and machines, the air pierced by beeps and alarms.

The room had a narrow bench with a foam pad that we used as a couch during the day. At night it was a bed barely big enough for me. Kari slept with Emily, snuggling her close. These moments were precious, as she didn't know if she'd be able to do this tomorrow. Also, Kari wanted to feel Emily next to her to make sure that she was breathing.

As I struggled to sleep on the narrow bench, I thought about that little boy in the elevator. First, I thought, he was showing me that children are not weak in the way we adults assume they are. There's a lot they cannot do as children, but, when faced with something big like this, their spirits can be strong, and they can fight as hard as any adult. That was one lesson from the little boy.

The other thing that stuck with me was a question: Where were his parents? He'd seemed calm and self-possessed. I guess he'd been sick for a while and had developed this attitude to help him handle whatever came, but still I thought his parents should have been with him every minute of the time he had left. You take from these whispers what you feel strongly, and I felt strongly that boy was a sign that we should never leave Emily alone.

Late that night, a nurse's aide's panicked voice startled Kari awake.

"Emily! Sweetie!" the aide said, shaking Emily gently on the shoulder. "Can you open your eyes for me?"

Emily didn't move.

"She's not breathing!" Kari said.

The aide pressed the code blue button and ran out of the room yelling, "I need help in here!"

I jumped up. Emily was limp, her eyes rolled back into their sockets. Her skin looked blue. As I bent over her to start CPR, the door flew open and a team of doctors and nurses rushed in.

"We're going to have to bag her," a male nurse yelled.

He positioned a resuscitator over Emily's face to start pumping air into her.

A young doctor placed a stethoscope on Emily's chest.

"Start a second IV!" she ordered.

A nurse stuck an IV needle in Emily's foot, and she took in an audible gasp of air. Thank God!

We soon learned that Emily had too much morphine in her system, which had suppressed her breathing. The attending physician ordered Narcan, a medication for drug overdoses. After the Narcan, Emily's breathing regained its rhythm. Everyone in the room relaxed as we watched her oxygen level steadily increasing on the monitor. One by one the staff filed out, satisfied the situation was under control.

Kari and I sat on the bench, holding hands and unable to speak. We were shocked and terrified that we had almost lost Emily when we had been right there.

Chapter 2

OUR NEW REALITY

The light of dawn coming into Emily's hospital room surprised Kari and me. We hadn't slept at all and had lost all sense of time. The doctor on call came in to apologize and explain that the morphine pump had malfunctioned. They switched Emily to morphine injections every two hours, and they agreed to my request to transfer us to a bigger room.

In the new room, which had a window facing the woods, Emily lay in the bed with her arms extended, pricked by IV lines. She was monitored by a multitude of sensors that made soft blipping noises. Kari was tucked into a curl in an armchair near Emily's bed, poring over a thick book about leukemia that the hospital social worker had given us. *Childhood Leukemia: A Guide for Families, Friends, & Caregivers* by Nancy Keene was written for parents whose children had just been diagnosed, and I could hear Kari flipping through the pages, absorbing every word. This was the way Kari handled her fears, by trying to learn more and to understand better. Me, I was looking out the window and praying.

I stood at the window looking at the woods on the other side of the parking lot. Everything was moving so fast, but we were in a kind of parental limbo. We understood how dire the situation was but could do nothing to make it better. I wanted to take charge, to make decisions to save my little girl's life, and I knew that Kari felt that way, too. But until Emily got more tests, and we knew exactly what type of leukemia she had, there wasn't anything to do.

I remembered the binoculars sitting at the top of my duffel bag and grabbed them. I scanned the woods looking for deer, or a flock of turkeys, so I could take refuge in the natural order of things. In the natural order of things, Emily would survive, and she would outlive Kari and me. We would be back at our family camp soon using these binoculars to chart the flight of a bald eagle, or the scampers of a squirrel. This was why these binoculars had whispered to me when I was shoving things in the car back at the house.

I heard Kari close the book and I went over to be next to her and to ask her what she'd learned beyond what the doctors had told us. I always think of cancer as a tumor in tissues, like breast cancer or lung cancer, but I learned that leukemia is a blood cancer.

With leukemia, the bone marrow overproduces immature white blood cells, called blasts, which never mature enough to fight infection. These ineffective blasts multiply rapidly and crowd out red blood cells and platelets. Red blood cells carry oxygen throughout the body. Emily's red blood cell count was low and she was anemic, which was why she was tired and looked so pale. Platelets are the cells that form blood clots to stop bleeding. Emily's platelets were dangerously low, which is why she bruised so easily and her gums bled when she brushed her teeth. Without healthy white blood cells to fight viruses and bacteria, Emily was extremely susceptible to infection. The doctors suspected she had acute lymphoblastic leukemia, or ALL, the most common type of cancer in children. As Kari read in the book, ALL is considered to be the most curable childhood cancer because approximately 90 percent of children treated for it are alive five years later and considered to be cured.

"These are pretty good odds," I said.

"They are," Kari said, but her face didn't show that she felt optimistic. "I thought there would only be a few months of treatment, but the book says treatment takes more than two years."

We sat for a moment and let that sink in.

"Why is this happening to Emily?" Kari cried.

"There's no sense in asking that question or saying, 'Poor us.' I don't want Emily to feel like a poor little sick girl. We have to be strong for her," I said. "I was thinking, 'What do I want Emily to feel like?' I want her to feel we're going to beat this. We're going to be strong and we're going to beat it."

Kari's phone rang and she just looked at it. The whole time we'd been talking, I had felt mine vibrating in my back pocket. News of Emily's illness had lit up Philipsburg's grapevine. I grabbed my phone and saw messages and missed calls from my brothers, my cousins, and friends I'd known since elementary school. I showed the screen to Kari, and she showed me the person calling her: Mom.

Neither of us had the energy to talk to anyone else.

"Tom, I failed Emily," Kari said. "I slept next to her so I'd know if she needed me. She did, and I didn't feel it. She could have died right next to me."

"Kari you will never fail her," I said. "You're doing everything you can."

My phone rang again, and I saw it was my brother Jim. I'd talked to him the night before. By the time the grapevine reached him, he was getting inaccurate information. He said people thought Emily had lymphoma, not leukemia. And Kari had a cousin who thought we were in the hospital because I was the one with cancer. How were we going to keep our family and friends informed without spending all day on the phone?

"I'm going to start a blog," said Kari.

"What?"

"The social worker told me about a website called CaringBridge where you can blog about a loved one who is sick," Kari said. "We can describe what is happening. Just the facts. For instance, today I will write about how we found out Emily was sick and how we ended up at Hershey. I can write exactly what is happening and then it's coming from me, coming from us, so they know what is accurate."

"Good idea," I said. "Just put the facts. Then everyone can read it instead of passing information from phone call to phone call. And they can leave notes or ask questions in the comments section."

"I'm going to start now," she said, opening her laptop.

"Are you hungry?" I asked. "I'm going to see what I can find for breakfast."

"Not now," Kari said, already typing.

I walked out into the hallway past the nurses' station toward the family lounge. Each of the doors I passed in the hallway had six small panes of glass. I could see the kids inside the rooms. I saw one child with her mom bent over the hospital tray as they colored together. This child had a lot of artwork taped outside her door, which made the hallway more cheerful, but I knew it also meant that that family had been in the hospital for a long time.

The lounge had a sitting area, a refrigerator where families could store food, a sink, and a microwave. I grabbed a piece of my mom's banana bread from the refrigerator. She'd stashed one of her famous loaves in the bag of snacks she'd put together for us to bring to the hospital. I took my breakfast and a cup of coffee to a table. Soon I was joined by an older woman, short and thin with neatly trimmed gray hair and fierce eyes, wearing sweats and a boxy T-shirt. Her eyes lingered on me as she gathered up juice and protein bars.

"You're new here," she said.

"We just arrived yesterday," I said. "How long have you been here?"

"Six weeks." She sighed, taking the seat opposite mine.

"You know, the parents on the cancer unit can get vouchers for cafeteria meals. Ask the nurses," she encouraged me, indicating the protein bars she held in her hand. "Eating this stuff is not good for you."

"Thanks," I said. "That's good to know."

She reached over and gave my hand a little squeeze before she stood.

"Welcome to hell," she said. "We're your companions on this unit and we support each other. Try to be kind to everyone you meet."

• • ✦ • •

When I got back to the room Emily was awake. Kari was in the bed next to her, helping her page through a book. Emily was subdued and wary, not herself.

We thought that taking her outside to enjoy the beautiful day would boost her spirits. We pushed her outside in her wheelchair, but she wanted to run; she wanted me to chase her. But she couldn't do any of that and started to cry. We took her back in right away. I think she was trying to wrap her mind around her illness and her new surroundings. Normally she's a girl with dozens of questions, but so far she hadn't asked many. Kari offered to take her to the playroom, where they had games and lots of art supplies, and T-shirts you could draw on, but she was embarrassed.

"I can't go like this!" she cried tearfully, holding up her arm with the IV in, even though we assured her that all the other kids there would have those, too.

Over the next few days some of our family stopped by to visit. Aunt Laurie brought her teenagers Meaghan and Nate, and Kari's sister Kristen and her fiancé, Nick, visited. When Kari's mom, Pam, or "Nana Pam," as Emily called her, came to visit, she encouraged Kari and me to take a break and leave the hospital for an hour or two.

We decided to drive to Target to pick up a few things, but once we were outside of the hospital, we understood why Emily felt so sad when we'd taken her out. The world seemed too bright and noisy, and oblivious to what was happening to us. People walked by chatting on their phones and laughing. Cars passed by blaring summer pop tunes. We felt like we no longer fit into everyday life. We quickly shopped for the items we needed and hurried back to the hospital. Emily cried when she saw us. She had missed us. We knew it would be quite a while before we did that again.

We were anxious for it to be Tuesday so we'd have a confirmed diagnosis. We signed the permission forms for the diagnostic tests on Monday evening so Emily could begin testing first thing in the morning. The nurses explained that once Emily started chemotherapy it would not be long before she started to lose her hair. Her hair was one of her best features: lustrous, thick, and chestnut brown. Kari had it cut at chin length for the summer, with straight bangs that framed her face beautifully. I didn't think that Emily would take it very well when it started to fall out. The social worker explained how some parents like to get their child's hair cut right after the diagnosis so that when it starts to fall out there will be only little wisps to brush away. It just so happened that local stylists volunteered to cut patients' hair at the hospital once a week and would be stopping by that day. The stylist gave her a cute, and very short, pixie cut.

I thought she looked adorable with her new haircut but Emily was furious. Kari was angry at me, too, because she thought I'd acted too quickly. She felt that we were taking something else away from Emily when she already had so little control over what was happening to her. But what was done was done. We had to focus on things that could make Emily happy, or at least distract her.

The thing that made Emily truly happy that day was a visit from Jasper, one of several therapy dogs that came around once a week. Jasper was a mutt with a shiny black coat. You didn't need a pedigree to help a child heal. The moment they met in the hallway outside Emily's room, her mood transformed. She loved Jasper and was so sweet with him. We were grateful her haircut happened to be on his visiting day.

———————— ··•·· ————————

On Tuesday morning, we met with Dr. David Ungar, who would be Emily's primary oncologist. He explained that two of the tests—the bone marrow aspiration and the lumbar puncture (also known as a spinal tap)—would be painful. Emily would have to be sedated to endure the long needles he would be using to get the samples from her. I could see how anxious it made Kari to think about Emily being in so much pain. After all I had experienced with Crohn's disease, medical procedures didn't scare me, and I wanted to be there for Emily. Dr. Ungar said it was okay for me to stay in the room while he took the samples.

I watched Dr. Ungar sedate Emily through her IV. He explained that Emily would be semiconscious during the procedure, but she wouldn't remember any of the pain she went through.

Dr. Ungar warned me that Emily might become emotional and say hurtful things as the medication started to take effect. I pulled a chair up to the exam table so I could be close to Emily and hold her hands in mine. He turned Emily on her side to face me. When the drug took effect, Emily was whimpering and crying softly. I watched Dr. Ungar insert a long needle into a blue plastic handle, gripping it between his middle and ring fingers, making a tight fist. He jabbed the needle deep into the saddle of her rear right hip, pushing and turning the handle until he felt the needle break into the bone. Emily's cries became louder when she felt the pressure of the needle.

"Why are you letting them hurt me, Daddy?" she whimpered. "Make them stop! Make them stop!"

"Everything's going to be all right," I said softly stroking her head. "This won't take long."

Next Dr. Ungar collected a sample of Emily's cerebrospinal fluid, probing her spine with his fingers to find the correct spot to guide the needle between her vertebrae. Her spinal fluid dripped into a small collection tube. The procedures were exhausting for Emily. She went right to sleep afterward and was still sleeping when we returned to the room.

Kari was making great progress on the blog. She'd already finished describing how we learned that Emily was sick and why we were at Hershey. She was just waiting for me to read it over before she posted it on the website. I appreciated the way Kari wrote, how she managed to express what was happening without getting corny or sentimental like I would.

I only wanted to add one thing, about the whispers. Kari wrote,

Everyone keeps saying "but she was healthy, she wasn't sick, was she?" No, she wasn't sick. She had plenty of energy, was eating great, wasn't losing weight. She seemed absolutely fine... until the little things I had started to notice began adding up.

I've heard Oprah say, "Listen to the whispers in your life." Yes,
I just quoted Oprah! But it really seems to apply here. Little things
I tried to ignore would become really important.

—Kari's journal

May 29, 2010

————••◉••————

When Dr. Ungar came into Emily's room to discuss the test results, he
had a smile on his face and spoke with confidence.

"As we suspected, Emily has standard-risk acute lymphoblastic leukemia. If your child gets cancer, this is the one to get, because we're very
good at treating this type of leukemia," he said. "It's what we call the
garden-variety type of leukemia. It is the most common and most curable
cancer in children. After Emily goes through treatment, she'll have a long
life ahead of her. She'll grow up to be a grandmother."

I thought this was an odd thing to say, but it must have been his way
of preparing us for the scary numbers he was about to share from the tests.

The bone marrow aspirate showed that 99 percent of the cells in Emily's bone marrow were leukemia cells. Thankfully, there were no cancer
cells in her spinal fluid, which would have made the cancer more difficult
to treat. She would be treated with chemotherapy to wipe out the cancer
cells and make room for the bone marrow to make healthy cells again.
The treatment would take two years and two months.

More than two years of chemotherapy? Kari and I looked at each
other. That felt like a lifetime.

For the next month, Emily would be in the first phase of treatment
called the induction phase. The goal of this phase was to get Emily into
remission—meaning to eliminate most of the cancer cells. She would get

IV chemotherapy once a week and take chemotherapy pills daily. The drugs would destroy all her blood cells—not only cancer cells, but also any healthy cells—suppressing her immune system. We had to be careful not to expose her to germs, which meant limiting the time she spent with other people. She would also need blood and platelet transfusions, sometimes several a week, until her bone marrow started producing healthy cells again. Emily would be in the hospital for this first week, but after that we could go home, returning to Hershey weekly for outpatient chemotherapy.

After that would be the six-month consolidation/intensification phase, where they would give her different combinations of chemotherapies to kill off any remaining cancer cells. Emily would be admitted to the hospital several times during those months for inpatient chemotherapy. If all went well, the doctor explained, the last phase was maintenance, when Emily would get chemotherapy once a month at the outpatient clinic. During each phase, she would also take chemotherapy pills, pills to keep her from contracting a certain type of pneumonia, pills for nausea, and pills for pain—up to seventeen pills on some days. In addition, anytime she ran a fever higher than 100.5 degrees, we had to take her to the emergency room for IV antibiotics or she risked getting sepsis. With her suppressed immune system, any infection could get out of control quickly.

The nurse handed us a schedule outlining which medications Emily would need each day, a schedule that she said would change every month depending on how Emily's treatment was progressing. It was overwhelming and daunting to keep track of.

The good news was that we could be home as early as Sunday if she adjusted well to this first round of chemotherapy. Another piece of good news was that Dr. Ungar didn't see any reason to postpone kindergarten, which Emily was supposed to start at the end of the summer. She would miss some school during the more intense weeks of chemotherapy, but there was no reason to delay.

Kari and I were worried about how sick the chemotherapy would make her and the suffering that she would go through. Yet we were happy to hear that Emily could begin school. We also liked that we had a plan to follow and we knew what to expect.

We were also surprised by the big audience that was responding to the blog. One of the ways we could boost Emily's spirits was to read her some of the comments from all the people who wished her well, some of whom we didn't even know. Our families and our friends had shared it with their families and their friends. Everyone in Philipsburg seemed to be following it, and a few people in different states as well.

A few hours later, one of Emily's favorite nurses, Nurse Karli, came in to follow up on how we were understanding the diagnosis. Nurse Karli is blond and petite like Kari, and she was funny as well as beautiful, with a spirit that matched Emily's. She was always trying to make her patients laugh. But on this visit, Nurse Karli was not joking around. We saw her tender side.

Nurse Karli gave Emily a booklet called *The Story of the Bone Marrow Bandit*, which she'd made for another patient with leukemia whose name was Edda. The first drawing was a cross section of a bone—Edda's bone marrow cell factory—identifying the red blood cells, white blood cells, and the platelets. Outside the factory hung a big sign announcing that it was hiring: "White Blood Cell position available—inquire within."

The other cells were busy doing their jobs when a not-so-nice white blood cell named Lymphocyte was hired. Nurse Karli described him as "young and immature and never did his work properly." Then he invited his other blast friends over to his cozy spot, and they invited their blast friends, too. With so many of these loafers crowding out the productive cells, the blood cell factory had to shut down.

This simple way of describing leukemia really got Emily's attention. She looked keenly at Nurse Karli's drawings.

These lazy, immature white blood cells caused a panic in the organs, which started asking each other what was going on. The lungs were tired and, without fresh platelets, suddenly Edda bruised easily. Edda went to a special doctor, Captain Chemo, who brought in strong medicine. Nurse Karli drew Captain Chemo as a drop of medicine with its fists on its hips, chin high and wearing a cape, ready to kick out the lazy blasts.

Nurse Karli had given us an avatar—Captain Chemo—the hero medicine that would take Emily's cancer away.

After Nurse Karli left, Emily didn't want to draw or read. I could see that the wheels were turning in that little head of hers. Through Captain Chemo, she better understood what was up ahead, and she was thinking that through.

The setting sun hit the woods across the parking lot at a low angle, sending broad shafts of light through the trees. I wondered what Emily and I could see if we took a look at the woods. There were always moments when I wanted to take her out of this.

"Emily, the forest over there is glowing," I said, picking up my binoculars. "Do you want to see what we can see?"

Kari helped her get to her feet and I steered her IV pole. When we got to the window, she took the binoculars and put her elbows on the windowsill to steady her arms as she scanned the woods.

"Daddy, there's a flock of turkeys running through those trees, and a squirrel! He's really fast up that tree," she said.

"Really?" I said. "Let me see!"

I crouched alongside her, and she offered me the binoculars. I saw the turkeys, and that gray squirrel going down a tree, and then up again. I handed them back to her.

When she put them back up to her eyes she gasped with joy.

"Daddy! I see a butterfly!" she exclaimed. "Even from all the way over here, I can see the butterflies in and out of the trees."

This was why I'd grabbed those binoculars. To show her that life outside this room was what we were aiming for, that that's what we wanted to get back to, going outside and doing things again. She had to know, and she had to see, that there was a world waiting for her outside this hospital room, and the world needed her in it.

Chapter 3

PLEASE PRAY FOR EMILY

It's scary being home. I feel like I need to disinfect the entire house so she doesn't get sick. Then I started worrying that the Clorox disinfectant I was using on the countertops was probably toxic and causes leukemia. I'm wondering if I should throw out all my cleaners and buy all-natural products. Then I gave Emily strawberries and worried that the pesticides used on them probably caused leukemia, too. I think I'll go to Wegmans tomorrow so I can stock up on all organic food.

—Kari's journal
June 5, 2010

After a week of chemotherapy, we brought Emily home, and it was amazing to watch Kari in action. She disinfected the house, bought all organic food, and made a master medication schedule and a chart to record Emily's temperature fluctuations and her daily routine. Before we left Hershey, Emily had a PICC line (peripherally inserted central catheter) inserted into a vein in her right arm to make it easier for her to get IV medicines and blood draws. We had to make sure that the insertion point in her arm didn't get infected. Kari was determined to notice any signs of infection as soon as possible.

That was why, after the joy of homecoming, we started to miss the security of the hospital. At Hershey, nurses swept in and out of the room to check on Emily, to adjust something, or to administer medicine. We never had to worry about Emily's pain because all we had to do was mention it and the nurses would make her comfortable. Nor did we have to be concerned about making it to a doctor's appointment. Now all of that fell on us, and we were anxious not to make a mistake.

Normally our house is full of visitors, with Emily's cousins dropping by and the other members of our families coming for dinner. We are very close with our families, and we already missed them. The fact that Emily could not see her cousins and that we had to restrict visitors was sad for her—for all of us, really.

A few days after we settled back in at home, I could see that Emily was discouraged, and it upset me. Since we needed to protect Emily from germs, the only thing I could do with her was drive by her cousins' house so she could see them out the car window as we passed.

She was excited to get into the car. I could see her in the rearview mirror squirming higher in her seat to look out the window when we turned onto the street where her cousins Ryan and Jeremy lived. She got a big smile on her face when we pulled up to their house. They knew we were coming and had been watching for us through the window. They rushed out, pounding down the front steps. I stopped the car for a few minutes, watching as Emily held her hand up to the window so that her cousins could hold up their hands to bump fists, as if they were giving her love through that pane of glass. I saw how her smile collapsed into sorrow when we had to pull away from their house, only reinforcing that so much was different since she got sick.

At home, the financial reality of our situation hit us. Although we had good health insurance, this was going to be more expensive than we could even imagine. The hospital bills and explanations of health benefits kept arriving in the mail, some of them dozens of pages thick, stuffed into large envelopes that we didn't want to open. It took all our energy just to make sure that Emily was doing okay. We both always wanted to be with her, but to keep some money coming in, we agreed, we'd each work part time. The heartfelt piece of this was how our community was starting to respond to Emily's illness.

We read Emily the comments on the blog every day and also set aside time for her to open the get-well cards that filled our mailbox. All over town, people we barely knew were keeping us in their thoughts, which we saw on the blog but also in other ways. Robin, Kari's dad, who Emily called "Pappy Rob," worked at a bank. He's a modest man who keeps to himself, and he's a man of very strong faith. I knew he was praying several times a day for Emily, but it was not something he'd talk to his coworkers about. And, although he didn't explain why he'd left the day she was diagnosed, when he got back to work he found an envelope with twenty dollars in it and a note that said *Good luck to your granddaughter.*

That twenty dollars meant so much. I knew deep in my bones that our small town and our families would always lift us up, and I had a feeling that the Lord would provide. That first twenty dollars coming so quickly showed I wasn't wrong to think that. As the audience for the blog grew, people in town or at church handed my parents gift cards for gas stations and restaurants.

Although most of Emily's treatment would be on an outpatient basis, we still had to make weekly trips to Hershey for her chemotherapy. For the first trip back to Hershey, Kari was going to work that day, so Pappy Rob volunteered to come along. Pappy Rob was scheduled to come to the house at 7:00 a.m. so we would have plenty of time to get Emily to Hershey by 11:00 a.m.

That night, around 2:00 a.m., Emily woke up screaming and I ran to her room.

"My legs," she shrieked. "There's something wrong with my legs!"

"Is it your knees?" I asked.

"No!" she pointed to a spot in her thigh. "It's there. It's right there."

I tried to pick her up, but she yelled at me not to. Kari heard Emily's cries and came in with some morphine to help with the pain. I paged Dr. Osman Khan, who had become one of our favorite doctors at Hershey. We always slept better when he was the doctor on call at night, and he always responded quickly when we called.

"Emily's screaming, in the most pain she's ever had. It's a ten out of ten on the pain scale and if I touch her, she screams louder. Do we need to bring her in?"

"Put her in the car and drive straight here." Dr. Khan said. "Give her three times the normal dose of morphine. She can handle that much."

I called Pappy Rob, with Emily screaming in the background, to tell him that if he wanted to come along, we needed to leave right away. He said he'd come immediately. As I was getting ready to go, Kari stopped me in the kitchen.

"I know what you are thinking," she said. "I know because she's in so much pain you're going to want to take her to the nearest hospital. Promise me you will not check her into Mount Nittany Medical Center. Whatever is wrong with her, she needs to be at Hershey."

We pass Mount Nittany Medical Center on our way to Hershey, and although it's a great facility, it doesn't have a pediatric oncology unit.

Emily would just end up in an ambulance ride or Life Flight to Hershey if we stopped there.

"Okay, I'll make sure," I said.

"Tom," she said sternly. "I want to hear you say it. I want you to look me in the eye and promise that you will drive straight to Hershey."

"I promise," I said.

Pappy Rob arrived and I went to pick up Emily to put her into the car.

"Don't touch me! Don't touch me!" she screamed.

"Look, Em," I said. "I have to get you into the car!"

We put pillows under her legs so she would be cushioned against the bumps in the road, and Pappy Rob sat in the backseat right next to her. The morphine didn't help the pain, though. She was screaming as we merged onto the highway near State College, right next to Mount Nittany Medical Center. Why should I make her endure the two hours it would take us to get her to Hershey when she was in this much pain? My poor girl. But I had made that promise to Kari and I wouldn't break it, despite what I felt.

"Daddy, I have to pee," Emily said softly. Then, more desperately, "I have to pee really bad!"

I couldn't take her into a gas station in the shape she was in. I couldn't take her into Mount Nittany because that would surely create a cascade of actions that would get her admitted there. I pulled over to the emergency room entrance and jogged inside, where I asked one of the nurses if he could give me a bedpan. He kind of cocked his head like a dog does when he hears a sound he doesn't understand. I told him he had to trust me on this. He came back with the bedpan and soon we were on our way. When we were nearly to Hershey, I called the oncology clinic to arrange for someone to help us get Emily out of the car. They said they would have someone meet us with a wheelchair.

When I saw the nurse standing with the wheelchair, I realized that bending Emily's legs to sit, touching them that much, would be torture. I put my hand on Emily's leg to move her and she started screaming.

"I'll get a bed instead," the nurse said, running back into the clinic.

In the examination room, I saw that her left thigh was swollen to twice the size of the right one. On that left thigh was a raised red mark about the size of a quarter. That hadn't been there when we left home two hours before.

I showed the nurse what I had discovered.

"I'll get the doctors right away," the nurse said.

A group of doctors came quickly. The senior one examined her wound and handed me a marker.

"Dad," the doctor said. "Take this marker and circle the red area. We're starting her on morphine and antibiotics. As long as the infection stays within that circle it means the infection is not spreading."

Pappy Rob and I were relieved to finally be in the hands of the people we trusted and grateful that Emily had stopped screaming. About twenty minutes later I checked her leg and saw the area had grown far outside the circle I had drawn, and the color had changed from red to purple.

I motioned the doctor over and he immediately ordered an MRI. I called Kari and told her she needed to get here right away.

"I'm on my way," Kari said.

They wheeled Emily into the MRI room and said they would sedate her because she might panic in the tube. This did not set well with Emily, who seemed to be on the edge of panic already.

"You're not leaving me, Daddy," she said.

"I'll stay here," I said. "Whatever it takes."

They gave her the anesthetic and, as she was slipping into unconsciousness, the last thing she said was "You still can't leave. Even when I'm asleep."

"Okay," I said. I was sitting there cradling her hand in mine and watching that her chest was still moving up and down. I was so scared that she was going to stop breathing again. At one point my Saint Christopher's necklace floated up from my chest toward the MRI magnet. I had to take it off and put it in my pocket.

When we came out of the MRI, Kari was there with Pappy Rob. We passed the surgical team assembled at the nurses' desk studying Emily's MRI. They talked in low voices, bumping each other out of the way as they debated what they saw there. Nurse Karli arrived for her shift. I told Nurse Karli I was worried that Emily's infection was something they'd never seen before and they might not know how to handle it. We needed the best surgeon they had, I insisted, not just whatever surgeon was on call. She pointed to the doctor who was trying to settle the discussion in front of the MRI.

"Tom, that's the chief of surgery, Dr. Dillon," Nurse Karli said. "He doesn't usually come here this late on a Friday." We knew it must be serious if the chief of surgery came in on a Friday night.

We went back to Emily's room, where Pappy Rob was sitting with our sleepy girl, who was still knocked out from the MRI. We'd been there only a few minutes when a nurse told us that Dr. Dillon wanted to see us in a consultation room. When we stepped into the hallway, Kari started sobbing.

"They're going to take her legs," she said. "They're going to take us into that room to tell us that they have to amputate her legs."

"I don't think that's what they are going to tell us. Let's try to stay positive," I said.

We sat down at a table facing Dr. Dillon.

"Cancer is not your biggest problem tonight," he said. "You need to save your daughter's life. From the MRI, it looks like the infection in her left leg is completely through her muscle and into the bone. If it's in the bone, I will have to amputate her left leg at the hip."

Kari gasped.

"We also see the infection starting in her right calf. If it's in the bone there, I'm going to amputate her right leg at the knee. Her immune system isn't strong enough to fight this, so if it's in the bone, this is the only solution we have."

I grabbed Kari's hand under the table. She was not sobbing at that moment. She was stricken.

"I'm sorry I have to tell you this," the doctor said. "You have to sign the consent for the amputations now. I won't have time to come to talk to you if we find infection in the bone."

I signed the consent forms with such a heavy heart. If they had to amputate, would Emily hate me for the rest of her life for signing her legs away?

Emily had woken up while we were consulting with the doctors. She was giddy from the medicines they administered to help keep her calm. It wasn't long before we were walking alongside her bed as they pushed her down the hallway to the operating room. She was laughing and pointing to the ceiling, catching her reflection in the big spherical camera lenses positioned along the hallway.

"Look, Daddy!" She giggled. "I can see myself! Hello, Emily! Emily's riding down the hallway in her bed!"

"Yes!" I said, taking her hand. "There's our Emily on every camera!"

This was life in the hospital. We could go from the heaviest sense of dread and worry straight to this kind of silly.

The door to the operating room swung open and Kari and I kept holding Emily's hands until the nurse told us this was as far as we could go.

The doors closed and we could see the doctors and nurses moving around on the other side of the frosted glass. Watching these dark figures moving beyond what we could understand was not helping us be strong for Emily. We walked back to Emily's room to wait for an update from the surgical team.

"You have to ask people to pray for Emily," I said to Kari. "You need to post on the blog right away. We need everyone praying for Emily."

I know that many people don't believe in the power of prayer, but good thoughts and good wishes are just as powerful when all of them come together. That was how Kari wrote it in the blog:

> Please, please, please pray for Emily. She has a life-threatening infection in her leg. In surgery now. Have to take out all affected muscle in at least one of her legs. It may have spread to the other leg. She will be in the hospital for a very long time and be very sick. Please do not call or text Tom's phone...we are waiting for the surgeons to call on that phone and give us updates.
>
> —Kari's journal
> June 11, 2010

After Kari posted the update, Pappy Rob went looking for a chapel where he could pray. Without Emily's bed in the room, we felt her absence as a huge hole in the middle of our lives. We didn't even turn on the lights as we sat there in silence. I tried to think how I would explain to her when she woke up why her legs were gone, but I couldn't imagine a way to start.

About an hour into the surgery two of the oncologists burst through the door into the room.

"We're going to save her legs!"

Kari and I hugged each other tightly, breathing huge sighs of relief.

When Dr. Dillon opened up Emily's legs, he'd seen that the infection was in the sac around the muscles, not in the muscles or in the bone. Emily would be out of surgery soon, the doctor said, but not out of the hospital for weeks. They would attach wound vacuums to her legs to suck out fluid to reduce swelling and infection. She would need surgery every forty-eight hours over the next two weeks to adjust the pressure in the wound vacs.

Who would have thought we'd be overjoyed that our daughter would need surgery on her legs every two days? But we were. "The prayers worked," I said. "It's because everyone is praying for Emily."

"We're never splitting up for these appointments again," Kari whispered.

"Never."

Chapter 4

ONLY WORRY WHEN THEY GO QUIET

I was standing at the end of Emily's bed in the pediatric intensive care unit (PICU) wearing her pink tutu over my jeans and holding big blue-and-white Penn State cheerleader pompoms. During our first stay at Hershey, I got Emily to agree that we needed to smile at least once a day. For that first stay, it hadn't been that hard. This second stay, she'd become an expert eye roller, but genuine smiles were a lot harder to get. Just the day before, when I reminded Emily of our goal, she shot me a perfunctory smile and said, "Is that enough?" It wasn't.

On this day, I thought my best chance to meet our goal was for me to don this getup. She and Kari were looking at me blankly, as if they couldn't wrap their minds around my outfit or didn't want to. So I moved on to the cheer.

"Give me an E! Give me an M! Give me an I! Give me an L! Give me a Y! What does that spell? EMILY!"

"Dad…stop." There went the eye roll, but still no smile.

In that original stretch at Hershey, right after we'd had her hair cut, Emily was so sad and angry with me for insisting on her hair being shorn that I would have done anything to make her laugh. The problem was that I was getting tired, and not just because the sleeping situation was not so great. I felt as though I was coming down with bronchitis. I asked my doctor in Philipsburg to send me an injection of strong antibiotics. I said that I'd find someone at Hershey to inject me. She agreed, and my mom brought it along on her next visit. I knew just who I wanted to give me the shot. I watched the door, hoping to catch Nurse Rob.

I think both Emily and Kari had schoolgirl crushes on Nurse Rob. He was tall and had broad shoulders, olive skin, deep blue eyes, and a square military haircut that accentuated his strong jawline. For a big guy, he had a surprisingly delicate touch. We felt safe around him with his steady, genial manner. He also liked to play pranks on the other nurses. He and Emily would fill syringes with water, then press the call button so that when another nurse walked in, they could squirt them. I knew Emily would love it if Nurse Rob was the one who gave me the shot.

When I saw Nurse Rob passing by Emily's door, I jumped up.

"Rob! I need your help," I said, and he paused at the doorway. I held up the box that contained the antibiotic shot. "I need a shot in my butt."

I said "butt"! Emily sat up as straight as she could in bed to watch. She had a little hint of a smile at the corners of her mouth and her eyes were bright.

"I don't know," Nurse Rob said. "I'm not supposed to administer medicine not prescribed here."

"I understand," I said. "It's just that I think I'm coming down with something and I can't be sick around Emily. My doctor sent this to me. See? It's a prescription."

"Okay," he said, taking an exaggerated look up and down the hallway, as if he was frightened someone might see him coming into the room. He winked at Emily and put a finger to his lips.

"But remember, Emily: I was never here," he said.

While Nurse Rob set up the syringe, I placed one hand on the foot rail of Emily's bed, and with the other I pushed my pants down a bit on the left side. Emily and Kari were grinning as wide as I'd ever seen.

"This is going to hurt, isn't it?" I whimpered.

"You bet it is," he replied, poking his hand around on my hip, searching for the place to stick me. Emily's eyes darted between my clownish terror and very serious Nurse Rob on the job.

"The skin back here is *really* tough!"

I grimaced in anticipation, contorting my face like I was about to cry, while Nurse Rob took a huge swing with his arm to plant the shot in my backside. I watched Emily's head swivel to follow the needle on its way to the depths of my hip. Once it landed, I yelled and limped around, whimpered that he'd injured my leg. I moaned and wailed to the sky for forgiveness. Emily and Kari laughed so hard! For several days after that all I had to do to make Emily laugh was put my hand where Rob had stuck me and let out a moan.

Another surefire way to make Emily laugh was poop jokes. It seemed like the doctors always needed another stool sample. That's what no one talks about when they describe the way it is with families when a child gets sick. My family of three was tight and cozy, but we'd never had to be living in one room together for days on end. We became keenly aware of the way each other's bodies functioned, but most of the focus was on Emily. At first Emily was a little self-conscious producing these samples on cue. One of my fatherly bonds with my sweet little girl was poop humor, the kinds of jokes that disgusted or annoyed Kari. In some ways I think that made us laugh harder. When the doctors needed her urine, we would make a bet before she went to the bathroom. Whichever one of us guessed closest to the amount of urine she produced won. Right away we discovered an ally in Nurse Karli.

In the cancer unit they called Nurse Karli the Poop Nurse. Nurse Karli had jokes and games all designed to make children relax and let go. She was a specialist at potty humor. Some of her favorites were "What's brown and sits on a piano bench? Beethoven's Fifth Movement," and "Why are their only 239 beans in Irish bean soup? Because if you add one more it would be two farty."

She also used her Poop Nurse tools to help me teach Emily how to take her pills. Emily had to take pills several times a day, and some kids had trouble with that. I was determined that Emily would not be among them. I have had to take a lot of medicine for my Crohn's, so I know that choking down pills is unpleasant, but it's something you just have to get done. No grousing. I practiced with Emily, teaching her how to consciously relax her throat so she could swallow the pills, but we were still struggling. Nurse Karli saw what we were up to and offered Emily a reward for successfully taking her medicine.

"This is my deepest, most secret, high-level, pediatric oncology weapon," she said, holding up her cell phone with the Fart World app displayed on the screen. "If, when I come by on my morning rounds, your parents tell me that you've taken all of your medicines on time, you get to choose a fart."

Nurse Karli looked at the screen and chose Taco Truck, which let out a mighty sound. There were twenty choices on her app, ranging from Lima Beans to Echo Chamber.

"So, I'll be back tomorrow, and we'll see how it goes," Nurse Karli said.

"Nurse Karli! Nurse Karli, I took all my medicine on time today," I said. "Can I choose a fart?"

"Did he?" Nurse Karli asked Emily and Kari.

"He did!" Emily said.

I chose Jack the Ripper, which sounded like air slowly being squeezed out of the nozzle of a balloon. This got a big smile out of Emily.

Getting Emily to smile after the leg surgeries was a challenge because the wound vacs, one on her left thigh and another on her right calf, were extremely painful. Every day of my life I will be grateful that the doctors didn't have to amputate her legs, but the wound vacs were torture for Emily.

The wound vacs were made to fit into the wound on each leg. The nurses handcut a special piece of foam that they nestled snugly into each open wound, covered by a thin suction cup, which they secured with medical tape. A drainage tube came out from under the suction cup and connected to a portable vacuum pump. The wound vacs stood up plump on her slender legs, like little footballs. The vacuum sucked out fluid from the wounds and alleviated air pressure, which speeds up healing.

The nurses came into Emily's room several times a day to make sure the vacuums were gathering enough fluid. Turning the wound vacs off and on grabbed at those tender nerves in her legs, causing Emily tremendous pain. She trembled whenever a doctor or nurse entered the room, anticipating the pain they were about to inflict. She was so sensitive to anything touching her legs that she couldn't even tolerate being covered by a sheet. It was brutal for Kari and me to see her in so much pain.

Emily was also on steroids, which made her moody and bossy. The first day the steroids kicked in she ordered us out of her room. I forget what we did that displeased her, but she surprised us both when she extended her arm, pointed to the door, and said firmly, "OUT!"

We stayed in the hallway until she summoned us back in. Some days she gave us several "time-outs" a day. On those days I wished that Jasper, the therapy dog, was an on-call service animal, because every time he visited the oncology unit her mood changed to tenderness, at least for a while. It was a pity Jasper came only once a week.

After spending almost a week in the PICU, Emily was transferred back to the oncology unit. It was great to be back on the cancer floor. I never thought I'd say that! When we walked in, greeted by the oncology nurses we'd come to like and trust, it felt like a homecoming. Nearly having Emily's legs amputated changed our perspective. We hadn't thought anything worse than cancer could happen to Emily, but the leg infections made us realize cancer introduced many more problems than just the disease.

I was thinking a lot about how getting sick was shortening her childhood. Emily had always known her own mind, had strong preferences, and hadn't been shy about sharing her thoughts. Being the proud dad, I saw these qualities as marks of a leader. With the illness, we'd seen how she trained that energy on supervising her own care. We watched her become tougher, better educated. When a new nurse showed up, she paid closer attention. Any misstep got a sharp rebuke from Emily. When a nurse fumbled a step in accessing her PICC line Emily barked, "You should be fired! Bring in someone who knows what they are doing!"

I was pained to see that she was so attentive at a time when most kids don't have to worry about a thing. I made such a fool of myself at her bedside with pompoms in a bid to bring a little bit of that childhood back. I'm a really bad dancer and I can always make it worse. I was twirling around, shaking my butt, and failing at doing the splits.

"Hey, ya know? I'm pretty good at this," I said. "Maybe I should try out for the squad next year."

"Oh, stop," she said, with a small smile.

She was giggling—no sweeter sound in the world—when my mom arrived.

I pretended to trip and fell into a chair. Big smile accomplished.

"Oh, Tom, what are you doing now?"

My mom, Sandy, is only five feet four inches tall and is dwarfed by her husband and three sons, all of whom stand taller than six feet. People remember her as taller than she is because of her big heart. She's always thinking how to help someone, noticing people going through a tough time and bringing them a casserole. She also brings baked goods wherever she visits. As a nurse, the part of that job where she excelled was in supporting the best possible outcome, praying for it, and helping you see it when you couldn't see it for yourself. With my mom there, laden down with bags of snacks, books for Emily, and banana bread, I left to take a break down at the family lounge.

After only a few weeks in the hospital, I felt like an old-timer, and I knew why that grandma I met on the first weekend recognized me as a newcomer. I saw in the new parents the look we had had, that look of shock, and the thousand-yard stare of people who have not yet comprehended the magnitude of the change that has just occurred. I could also understand the wisdom of what that grandma said about being kind to everyone you met. I appreciated something else, too. The exchange I had with that grandma for maybe a minute was one that I would never forget. And, like that little boy in the elevator at Johns Hopkins, I knew I most likely wouldn't see her again.

Grandparents were the secret power behind the families in the pediatric oncology unit. The parents were on the front lines, and the grandparents provided logistical support. We could depend on them to bring stuff back and forth from home. My dad, Big Jim, who had a hard time traveling because of an injured back, had taken over our finances, paying our bills for us so when we went back home we wouldn't find that the cable was shut off. Kari's mom, Nana Pam, was so eager to see Emily that, whenever she got the chance, she literally ran through the hospital parking lot to Emily's room, always with a bag of books and some new crafts to share. She never talked to Emily about her illness; she just kept her busy.

Pappy Rob's approach was to keep her focused on helping others, making her the teacher. He told Emily he'd never been very good at drawing and she was, so he wanted her to teach him. They'd draw for hours with her gently critiquing his work, telling him to make the pants higher on SpongeBob SquarePants, or that the roof of the house was too big for the walls. The next time he visited, he'd pretend that he'd forgotten what he learned and ask her to start all over again with the houses and the trees. Emily never lost her patience with him, and I know she liked being in charge. Eventually, with the same spirit that had made her start giving us time-outs, she told him that he needed to address her by her teacher name, "Miss Em."

Among the gifts my mom brought that day was a little velvet drawstring bag.

"I got something for you," she said to me. "It's something for Emily, but it's for you, too."

She pulled open the satin cord around the top of the bag and pulled out two cloths that she draped over the foot rail of Emily's bed. They were healing cloths with an image of Jesus with a lady kneeling behind Him reaching out to touch His robe with the caption:

As many as touched the hem of His garment were made well.

Matthew 14:36

"A woman who had been bleeding for twelve years touched the hem of Jesus' cloak and instantly she was cured," Mom said. "It's in Matthew 9. He said to the woman, 'Take heart, daughter. Your faith has healed you.' Take heart, Emily. Your faith will heal you."

Mom reached into the pouch again and produced a small bottle of holy water and another of holy oil.

"This is holy water from Lourdes," Mom said. "And *this* is holy oil from Medjugorje, blessed by those children who had the vision of the Blessed Virgin. Our friends Rusty and Kristine had a healing with this oil, and they wanted me to bring it to Emily."

"Well, thanks, Mom," I said and hugged her, but I could see the amused look on my scientist wife's face as I gathered up these things and put them back in the bag. "Emily needs everybody to pull for her all the time."

Despite Kari's skepticism, we did believe we needed all the help we could get. That night when they almost had to amputate Emily's legs, Kari had posted "Please pray for Emily" on the blog, and people had. One friend texted me that he didn't sleep the whole night after he read that because he was so upset for Emily and the only thing he knew to do was to pray for her, all night. I heard that—or, as Kari would say, I *believed* I heard that, in the form of the whispers. The darkness of that room with the empty space where Emily ought to have been was filled for me with the sentiments of all the people who'd read about what we were facing and were praying and hoping and believing that it was going to be all right. And it was.

That night when the nurses came in to adjust her wound vacs, Emily was angry with them.

"All you do is come in here and hurt me!" she screamed.

She was screaming in pain, and yelling for them to stop, but the nurses had to finish the job.

"Emily, you're doing so well," I said, once the nurses were done. I sat holding her close. "You have to be brave. You have to stay strong."

"You keep telling me to be brave," she said to me with fury. "I'm not brave!"

"You know, Em, they only pick the bravest kids to fight cancer," I replied.

"You keep saying that. It's not true!" she said. "I'm not brave. I'm scared. It scares me every time the nurses come in."

"You know people who are called heroes have done something heroic in their lives," I said. "They were scared for their lives when they did it. Being scared means you're human. It doesn't mean you're not brave. You're brave because you keep fighting."

"No! It's just too hard!" she yelled.

I felt her tiny body relax into mine and knew she was on the edge of sleep. The screaming and pain had taken so much out of her.

"I don't care if I get better," she whispered in a voice not meant for anyone to hear. "They're not doing this to me anymore."

When we were sure she was asleep, Kari and I huddled close, because now we were scared. We had taken Emily's gumption and determination for a given. We had never heard her say something like that, and if she was shutting down, we thought it would be tough to get her back.

We agreed that we'd ask for a consult from a child psychologist. Emily had plenty of reasons to be upset. If she needed help mentally, I didn't want to be that stubborn dad who thought an encouraging word or her parents' love was enough. Psychology was not my thing, but then neither were prayer cloths.

One of the senior psychologists, Dr. George Blackall, came to see us the next day. He happened to come at a time when Emily was in a good mood. No one had fussed with her legs in hours and her pain was under control. She was coloring quietly, and we had music on for her. Kari was writing on the blog and I was looking out the window. Our new domesticity in the hospital.

Dr. Blackall motioned Kari and me out into the hallway for a word.

"I just wanted to tell you one thing," he said. "Your daughter screaming is the best thing that can be happening. She's on steroids that affect her mood and when she's screaming, she's exercising her lungs. That helps keep them clear of fluid, and she's less likely to get pneumonia."

"She screams at anyone who enters the room now and orders them not to come in," Kari said. "I feel bad for the nurses."

"Ah, don't worry about that," the doctor said. "These nurses are used to handling children screaming out of pain and frustration."

"Yesterday, what made us ask for an evaluation was when she said she didn't care if she gets better," I said.

"She's still talking to you. She trusts you enough to let you know exactly how she feels," he said.

A nurse brushed by us to attend to Emily.

"Oh no!" Emily yelled. "Not you! Get out of my room!"

The doctor grinned at us.

"I don't worry about the kids fighting cancer until they go quiet," he said. "When they go silent on me, there's something going on in their heads that may be hard to fix. Screaming is perfectly normal. Let her scream her head off. None of the medical staff are going to take it personally. Okay?"

"She's fighting," I said.

"And she's in a fierce fight," he said. "It's the battle of her young life."

"That hurts! You don't know how to access my line," cried Emily. "Get me a nurse that does. You don't get to try again!"

"She's fighting," said Kari with a rueful look.

"Yes," said the doctor. "And she's doing as well as anyone could hope."

Chapter 5

YOU'RE IN CHARGE OF HOPE

The days in the hospital room were long during this second stay. We trusted the staff, and the doctors were treating Emily with the best care, both emotional and medical, so we didn't have any battles to fight, and that was a blessing. Emily's legs were slowly healing. No amount of screaming and yelling would make that go any faster. Whatever the day presented, we'd deal with it as it came. Was she hungry or thirsty? Was she in pain? Did she need to walk a few minutes to strengthen her legs? Whatever it took to get through the day so we could be there tomorrow.

It's not a rousing battle cry: "Let's get through today!" The pressures this new life created filled up all the space in that hospital room.

I spent several hours a day on the phone with the insurance companies. I'd get on the phone with one person and they'd want to continue the call at another time, after they gathered more information, but they never called me back. Then I couldn't get that same person back when I called again. I'd get someone else who would say that he wasn't familiar with Emily's case and asked if I could start from the beginning. I'd start off the day in a reasonable mood, thinking that a pleasant manner always gets you further with people than starting off ready for a fight, but that kindly approach rarely lasted very long. I would say, "I'm trying to save my daughter's life, and this is not a good use of my time. I know it is in network and you're going to pay it."

Those were the fights about medical procedures that had already happened, but there were also fights about things to come. The doctors would tell us they were going to give her an expensive medication next Tuesday, and I would start on trying to get it approved—hour after hour on the phone. "No" was always the first response.

"Well, she has to get it to save her life," I'd say. "So what do we do to get it covered?"

"The doctor has to send a pre-authorization to us and then it goes to a committee and they'll decide if it's covered."

"Does the committee meet before Tuesday?"

"No, it does not." So here we go again.

Some days I could feel the stress and pressure building in the room and I knew that was not good for Emily. Often she reflected our mood, and at other times she set that mood with her behavior. Sometimes when Emily would hear these conversations, she would remind me, "Remember, Dad. We need to stay positive and smile once a day!"

On days when I sensed we were upsetting her, I'd suggest we go to the playroom. I wasn't good at crafts, but we had something else going on, a little father/daughter rivalry at the air hockey table. One way to get her out of a bad mood was to trash-talk with her about how badly I was going to beat her the next time we faced off.

"I've been practicing my moves while you took a nap, Emily," I told her one afternoon as I lamely shifted my hips back and forth, pretending I was the smoothest player known to the world. "I'm going to be an air hockey legend by the time you get better. I'm gonna smoke you."

"You are not!" Emily said, sitting up in her bed, keen to compete with me. "I can beat you even when I'm in a wheelchair. Let's go right now."

"Okay! Okay!" I said, stretching my arms out, loosening up for battle. Then a nurse came in holding two big bags for the IV pole.

"Emily needs these two medicines," she said, hanging them on the IV pole and then checking them off on her chart. "I'll start with your antibiotic. And after that I'm going to start your anti-nausea medicine. It will take about two hours."

"Do we have to do it now?" pleaded Emily. "We were going to go to play air hockey."

"I'm sorry, honey," the nurse said softly. "We have to stick to the schedule for you to get better. You can play right after we give you the medicine."

Emily was frowning, but then her face brightened with insight.

"You know those two medicines are compatible?" Emily said. "You can hook them up at the same time and it will take half as long."

"I don't think so," the nurse said, as she connected the first bag to the IV line. "But let me go check."

The nurse returned to the room with a big smile on her face after consulting with the other nurses down at the nurses' station.

"Well, how about that, Emily!" the nurse said. "You were right, clever girl."

Kari was so conscientious about the blog, I really admired her for the support she got for Emily just by stating the facts. We never asked for anything from the people who were following our journey except for prayers. My dad thinks that's why people back home were so generous. Emily's illness even made it into the local weekly newspaper, which mentioned Kari's blog, and increased our following even more. It was beautiful to think that people we'd never met were praying for Emily. As I sat there fighting my darkness, I could visualize people I loved kneeling in prayer at Saints Peter and Paul's church in Philipsburg and in other churches in nearby towns. People in my union were donating their vacation days to me for weeks at a time so that I wouldn't miss a paycheck, and Kari's colleagues at Penn State were doing the same. Some of the people who donated to me worked for my company in other states and didn't know me from a stranger on the street. Here we were, in the hospital 120 miles from Philipsburg, and even farther from my coworkers at First Energy scattered around five states, but I felt in my bones those openhearted commitments of support. Through the blog and through my whispers, we were connecting to a current of energy to support our little girl, and every day I was grateful for that, even at the moments when Kari and I were irritated with each other.

Emily was sleeping and I was yelling softly at our insurance company. Not the big, screaming, listen-you-damned-bureaucrat voice but the low, menacing you're-not-going-to-win-this-shakedown one that is more appropriate in front of a sleeping child. I wasn't going to get any satisfaction from this call, and I hung up with a firm thumb to the End button. An uncomfortable silence settled over the room. It was not a calm silence, but of frustration. Kari had been typing a new blog entry when she slammed her laptop shut.

"Sometimes I don't want to write just the facts. Do you know what I want to write, what I actually feel? Cancer sucks!"

"You probably shouldn't write that in the blog," I suggested, raising my eyebrows in surprise.

"I'll write what I'm supposed to write," she said. "I'm just telling you that sometimes I want to write my true feelings, but you want me to write only positive things. I want to say that we're watching our daughter endure horrific pain and that she's being burned from the inside with toxic chemotherapy. Not only are we watching our daughter suffer, but we listen to the other kids through these walls crying out in pain. I want to tell them how this feels like a nightmare from which we cannot escape."

"And we have no control over the schedule. They say she's getting a treatment at ten and then nothing happens until noon and we don't know how much time we're supposed to fill up before they take her. When are they going to come to take Emily to physical therapy?" I asked.

"It was supposed to be an hour ago," Kari said, exasperated.

"How are we supposed to know when to get her ready? I mean, she's sleeping!" I said, simmering with anger and ready to take it out on the next person who came along.

I sensed someone at the door. It was Nurse Karli. Who knew how long she had been standing there? She went to Emily, going through her routine of checking her vitals and consulting her chart. Something about the brusque way she entered the room chastened Kari and me, like she had caught us doing something we were not supposed to be doing.

Nurse Karli looked up from checking Emily's IV lines.

"I know I'm stepping outside my bounds to say this, but I'm going to say it anyway," Nurse Karli began. "You have to take care of your marriage."

We had nothing to say.

"I see it all the time here. Cancer takes a horrible toll on a family and if your marriage has any weaknesses, it's going to break it apart. You two need to remain strong. Many marriages don't survive a child's cancer, and then the child suffers even more," she said. "If you are fighting and angry and if your communication breaks down, then she starts missing appointments, and then you start fighting about that. You need to be a team, or it will get worse for her. You know how much she needs both of you."

I thought Kari and I were doing pretty good, but I also knew Nurse Karli had our best interests in mind.

"Do you have someone coming to visit today?" she asked.

"My dad's coming around six p.m.," Kari said.

"Well then, you guys are going out on a date."

"We can't leave Emily," I said.

"He's right," Kari said. "It scares her when we leave."

"You're going out on a date," Nurse Karli insisted. "I know this great little Italian restaurant, Fenicci's of Hershey, only a few blocks' walk away, where the owner takes great care of every couple I send his way. You better tell your dad, Kari. I'm going to go make a reservation for you at six thirty tonight."

Gotta love that Nurse Karli. Sometimes people have to take you by the shoulders and shake you to wake you up, and it takes a lot of courage to do that.

As six o'clock approached, the room was very busy. Miss Em was sitting up straight and alert, with art supplies close by her bed, and a few special items she'd asked her mom to get from the bag where they stored the scissors and stickers and such. Kari was doing something or other in the bathroom that was taking a pretty long time. At six on the dot, Pappy Rob arrived clutching the tablet he drew on and another bag of supplies from the art store.

"Miss Em, your student is here," he said, waving to me.

"And you're right on time!" said Emily. "Here, sit down right here."

"I was trying to practice since the last lesson but I think I forgot some of what you taught me," he said.

Pappy Rob opened his notebook to a page with some half-drawn houses.

"See, I was pretty good with the walls and what you taught me about the roof, but I wasn't so great at these windows," Pappy Rob explained.

"That's okay," Emily replied. "We can start all over from the beginning and we can spend more time on the windows."

"You know, Miss Em, you got me thinking about the windows," Pappy Rob said. He fished something out of the art store bag. "I thought maybe we could put glitter in them so they would look different from the rest of the house."

"Oooh!" Emily exclaimed, taking the glitter sticks in hand. "And we can fill the sky around the house with glitter, just like the stars! Thank you, Pappy."

The bathroom door opened and there stood Kari, beautiful as the day we met. She had fixed her hair and done her makeup, and she was wearing a necklace I gave her. We were going on a date, and she wanted to make it special. I loved that and I loved her beauty. Not just how beautiful she looks, but the beauty that comes from within her and touches everything she does.

Fenicci's was only a few blocks away and it was a pleasant summer evening, so Kari and I decided to walk there.

I took her hand. I'm not much for romantic gestures, but I have learned a lot about this part of life from Kari.

When we met, I was lightly attached to the world, thinking I hadn't much of a future. I'd just received the difficult news about my Crohn's disease from the doctor who said there wasn't anything he could do for me. I'd sought out that specialist at Johns Hopkins, and when Kari and I met, I'd just had that surgery. My life was just my illness. I would go to work and come home exhausted, spending most of my time at home. I wasn't interested in dating until I knew if I was going to live, because I didn't think it was fair to court a girl with the possibility of a marriage when I didn't know if I would be alive in a few years. Then Amy, a friend of mine from high school, said she had a stepsister she thought I'd like. I was just starting to think I might survive this disease, so I gave this a shot.

It was an old-fashioned situation. I had to go meet her family and spend some time with them before we could go out on our date. Stepping into that house was entering a different world. Kari's parents had split up when she was in high school, and Pam had raised her four girls for seven years before she'd married Kari's stepdad. Even with a man living there, it was still a house of women: neat and cozy, full of good meals, girlish laughter, and quiet secrets. This was the opposite of my childhood, with my dad and two brothers and my mom trying to hold her own in a sea of testosterone. Where the Whiteheads were big, rowdy, sarcastic, and always trying to pull a prank, Kari's home was polite and appropriate.

Thankfully, I didn't know what a big buildup my friend had given Kari. Amy told them I was a nice guy with a good job and who had a big family in the area. Kari had just broken up with a guy she had been dating since high school, and her sisters instigated this matchmaking because they were tired of Kari hanging around the house studying all day, but I think most of them still missed Kari's former boyfriend. Kari's sister Kristen, who is closest to her in age, looked at me skeptically when I stepped into the house. Her younger sisters, Brenda and Lindsey, who were in their early teens, took their cue from their mom, who liked me right away.

Kari and I went to see the movie *Good Will Hunting* and then I took her out to dinner. Amy had warned me that it would be hard to get Kari to talk because she's very reserved, but I didn't experience that. She had plenty to say, and she was a great listener. I always had more to say than she did, but she didn't mind that.

Even though I was not looking for love, I couldn't get her out of my mind in the weeks after we met. I wanted to take her to Sunday dinner to meet my family.

Back then, my mom made Sunday dinner every week for her sons and their girlfriends and any other members of the extended family who wanted to drop by. These dinners were noisy. My brothers and I were always teasing each other, insulting each other, telling terrible stories (many of them lies), and getting in pretend fights. Sometimes it could get crude. I could see the shock on Kari's face as the evening began and I think she went from shock to numbness at about the halfway point of the meal because the contrast between our home and hers was so overwhelming.

When everyone was done eating and joking, I grabbed some paper plates and started loading them down with dinner for my great-uncle and great-aunt, who lived across the street but were too ill to come to Sunday dinner anymore. I also fixed a plate for my grandma, who lived a few blocks away. My custom was to drop by for a visit with these dinners and sit awhile to see how they were doing and find out if they needed anything. I asked Kari if she wanted to come along, or if she wanted me to drive her home first. To my surprise, she said she'd really like to come with me. I did not know that she found my connection to family very attractive. Score one for me!

"Your family dinners…they're so different from mine," she said.

"I bet that's so," I said.

"I mean, your brothers tell crude stories, and they swear," she said. "That would never happen in our house."

"Well, boys versus girls," I said. "Can't deny the difference."

"And then you brought dinner to your aunt and uncle and your grandma," she said.

"Yes," I said. "I never miss a week unless I'm sick."

"And all I could think was, *What kind of person does this?*" she said. "It's so kind."

It's hard to express how happy she made me then. If she liked my family, and I liked her, that was pretty much all that I needed for us to continue on and see what happened. I knew it would be much harder for me, though, because I still had to impress Robin.

Kari's dad is a big guy, just like me, and he's protective of his daughters. Even after the divorce, Robin kept a close watch on his four girls. He was the kind of dad who, if one of his daughters was at another girl's house for a sleepover, might show up around midnight to make sure everything was as his daughter had described.

It took Robin more than a year before he stopped calling me Kari's friend and advanced me to the category of boyfriend. I guess I had to earn my way in, and it didn't always go smoothly. While I was angling for boyfriend status, I once made a huge mistake that set me back a few months.

We were out to dinner, along with Kari's sisters. I wanted to show Robin that I was making money and could support his daughter well. When I went to the bathroom, I sneaked over and picked up the check, proud of myself for the gesture. But it backfired. He was offended, because he pays for his girls when they are together, and I had stepped on that.

By the time I was officially Kari's boyfriend, Robin and I had had many long talks at his house while I enjoyed his superb grilled chicken and macaroni salad. He and I had become friends, and I was admitted into the family.

One of our more memorable dates was when I took her up in a little two-seater plane. I had started learning to fly the year before I met her, and Robin had cautioned Kari never to get up in a plane with me. She yearned to do it, though, and she finally agreed. I knew then that I wanted to ask her to marry me. I decided I'd ask her if she survived the flight!

We flew northwest from Philipsburg over the Moshannon State Forest, a place that had been rescued from disaster by the love of land in our community. In the 1800s the lumber barons clear-cut this beautiful land, leaving only stumps, decimating the wildlife, and encouraging erosion and fire. In the beginning of the 1900s, people saw this error. The state bought up the land a piece at a time, and gradually restored the forest. Although I'd never say something this sentimental to Kari, then or now, she had reclaimed me, too. When I met her, I was a man who didn't see his future, but with her at my side, I saw it clearly. We were well suited to each other in the way that our strengths and weaknesses nestled perfectly together. We also both loved the place where we were born. It seemed perfect to me to be swooping over the beauty of western Pennsylvania when I decided to ask her to marry me. A few days later, I purchased an engagement ring, bought red roses, cooked her dinner, and asked her to be my wife.

A decade later, on our date night in Hershey, we walked hand in hand into Fenicci's, and the owner, Phillip Guarno, treated us like family. It turned out that his daughter had had neuroblastoma, a cancer of the nerve cells, most common in infants. His daughter was better now, but he and his wife, Kveta, had been through what all the parents on the cancer unit were going through, and he wanted to give them the best time he could offer when they managed to get away from the hospital.

They sat us in a beautiful booth at the best vantage point in the restaurant and brought us appetizers on the house. It was a comforting room with soft lighting and hushed voices. As I looked at Kari in this light, it did feel like a date, and we were comfortable in a few minutes of silence that allowed both of us to let some of the stress fall away. Every time we'd gone away from the hospital before, all we talked about was the one subject that we thought about all the time: Emily. There didn't seem to be anything else as urgent. I didn't know how we'd answer Nurse Karli's challenge.

"We have to take care of our marriage," Kari said, echoing Nurse Karli.

"We do," I agreed. "It's the most important thing, after Emily."

"Sitting here, it feels hard to know where to start or what to do to make it better."

"I don't think we have to do much differently," I said. "Maybe what we're doing already is enough as long as we understand. Like you have a certain part of it that's yours and I am in charge of a different part, and in those areas, we never question each other's judgment. Sure, we talk about it, or maybe even joke about it, but we don't argue or second-guess."

"Well, you know me," she said. "I am comfortable in research. I want to read the research studies and talk with other parents about how treatment is going for their children."

"You know that world so well, Kari," I said. "You're thorough and when you tell me how you came to your opinion, I always admire how careful you are to consider everything you learned before you state what you think. And how you take notes on everything the doctors tell us. I trust you there, and I trust you on the blog, too. You're doing a great job there."

"Thank you. You know I want you to feel free to write, too," she said.

"I will once in a while, but I know you are doing it and I think there is something in you that needs to do it," I said.

"Yes. Some days seem so unreal," Kari said. "Putting down what happened every day, telling this story, helps me make sense of how one action leads to another. And the numbers—how her lab values fluctuate—the story that tells, too."

"These are your jobs. Perfect for you," I said. "What's left for me?"

"You're in charge of hope," said Kari with a smile.

I smiled back so wide. This *was* the perfect job for me. Being in charge of hope justified my terrible jokes and my stupid antics. Also, seeing as how hope was my job, I could handle pain with Emily in a way that Kari could not, because I could feel what was happening right then, but I had my eyes on the future when the pain was gone.

I was pretty pleased with our division of labor.

When we walked back to the hospital, we were more strongly connected than ever. We would fight in the future, of course, but our mutual respect and love were unquestionable.

That next day we got good news. The doctor said that when they took Emily in for her leg surgery they *might* be able to take the wound vac off the right calf. The left one, well, they weren't so sure about that one.

I wanted them both off so we could take Emily home. If the other wound vac remained on, we would have two more days with it on and then a few days after that to make sure the infection was gone, meaning at least another week in the hospital. That night after Emily fell asleep, I rummaged around in our stuff and brought out my mom's little drawstring bag that held the prayer cloths and the holy water and oil. Kari was looking at me from across the room with a sarcastic smile.

"Shhhhh!" I whispered to her. "I'm in charge of hope."

I rubbed a little holy oil on the prayer cloths and laid one on each of Emily's wound vacs. Then I walked down the side of her bed, sprinkling the holy water from Lourdes on her body and especially on her legs. For some reason this felt right to me. The next morning, I snatched the cloths away right before they took Emily off for surgery.

When they brought Emily back from surgery, she didn't have wound vacs on either leg. The doctor was amazed.

"It's always good to be proven wrong in this way," he said. "Her legs were doing so much better compared to yesterday when I examined them. She made a lot of progress overnight. We'll keep her a few more days to make sure there are no complications, but you might be able to be home by the weekend."

He thought *he* was pleased! I could barely wait to tell my mom.

Chapter 6

——··●··——

BACK HOME

Tom and I thought our lives were busy and stressful before we found out that Emily had leukemia...now we realize we had no idea what busy and stressful meant! Our days are filling up with doctor appointments, home nursing visits, physical therapy appointments, occupational therapy appointments...we have an appointment every day next week. I have no idea how we are supposed to go to work. Tom started back to work today while I stayed home with Emily.

—Kari's journal

June 24, 2010

It was June 23 before Emily was well enough that we could make the two-hour drive back to Philipsburg. Although I'd traveled US Route 322 between Hershey and home many times, this journey was much different. We had a new perspective. You know when you recognize that you are having a bad day and ask yourself, "Can this day get any worse?" We now had many examples that proved the answer to that question is yes.

The doctors said to us before we left that some children have a difficult induction phase. Emily's had been one of the most difficult they'd seen, but we had gotten through it. We were praying for fewer complications as we started the consolidation phase. The next step was to wait for her bone marrow to make new, healthy cells. We would go back to the oncology clinic in about a week, when Emily would get another bone marrow aspiration to see if she was in remission.

There had been such joy in Emily's hospital room as we bustled around packing up all the stuff we'd accumulated in the last two weeks. Some families liked to keep the rooms tidy. Compared to those people, we were a circus. Emily had at least a hundred get-well cards from friends and family that we had taped to the walls, and dozens of gifts. As we dismantled her room, we took all the cards off the walls and stacked the gifts in a big pile by the door. There were so many of them that we donated some to the oncology unit so that other kids could receive gifts. We had so much stuff that I had to borrow a cart from the hospital to get all of it to the car. It took several trips. I joked with Emily that I couldn't wait to get home and back to my man cave so I could watch HBO because we'd been watching the Disney Channel for weeks.

As we were packing, Kari suddenly remembered the Father's Day present she and Emily were working on right before Emily was diagnosed. Father's Day has always been special to me because that was the day Emily took her first step as a one-year-old. With everything that was going on, I hadn't even noticed that the Sunday before, June 20, had been that holiday.

Kari knew how much that day meant to me. Before Emily had been diagnosed, I'd known Emily and Kari were up to something, and I suspected it was about Father's Day. They'd kept going off together for hours, and they wouldn't tell me why or where they were going.

Sitting in the happy chaos of our dismantled hospital room, I found out what they'd been up to. Kari opened up her laptop to show me a video she'd made for Father's Day: a series of five photos of Emily holding up big letters she had made that spelled out "DADDY." It was the Emily of just a month ago, just a week or so before we found out she was sick. As I watched the photos slide by in a video, set to the song "Daddy-O" by Frances England, I cried. I was so grateful that Kari had captured these moments that we would always yearn for but could never come again. I took the video out to the nurses' station and showed it to them as a way to say farewell to the staff that had been so good to us for so long.

When all was ready to go, Emily asked if she could ride through the hospital on top of the last pile on the cart. Of course she could. We came down the hallway pulling the departing princess, and she smiled as she waved to everyone she passed on our way to the parking garage.

You know how when you have a long drive that you've done a bunch of times, you pick landmarks to note your progress? For me, we hadn't really left the grip of Hershey until we had crossed the Susquehanna River. The mood in the car always lightened when Emily pointed out the twenty-five-foot replica of the Statue of Liberty located in the Dauphin Narrows. When we reached the top of Seven Mountains, when it was literally all downhill from there, we were close to home.

I was thinking about my Father's Day present as I looked at Emily in the rearview mirror. I wondered how she would look to the people who hadn't seen her since she got sick.

I pulled off at the Philipsburg exit and drove past my brother Jim's house, past my grandparents' place, and into the driveway of our house, a few blocks from my brother Greg's. I expected both of my brothers would be dropping by that evening. Hell, when I knew we were at last coming home, I wanted to throw a big party and have everybody come to celebrate Emily. But Kari said no. Kari said we had to let Emily's wishes guide our actions. Maybe she would be tired or sick when we arrived.

Maybe she would be fine, just not ready for so much company right away. Kari was right.

I carried Emily up the stairs to our kitchen, and I could see my mom had been very busy anticipating our homecoming. The house was sparkling clean and the fridge was full of groceries, including a casserole for tonight, soup for tomorrow, and, of course, banana bread. I carried Emily down the hall into her room, where I saw mom's touch again. Emily told Nanny at the hospital that she missed her stuffed animals. Mom had arranged all one hundred of them in neat rows on the bed, grouped by animal, with her favorite stuffed lambs at the front. Emily pulled the lambs forward to set them in a semicircle facing her and Lammy, who had come with her to the hospital. Lammy addressed the assembled multitude from the crook of Emily's arm, explaining in a high-pitched voice littered with *baaaah*s how Emily and she had been to the hospital and it had been awful but now they were home, and they weren't going away again.

While we had been wrapped up in what was happening at the hospital, Emily's homecoming was front-page news in the Philipsburg weekly newspaper. There were cards from well-wishers in big bags on the kitchen table and, because so many people followed Kari's blog, dozens of "Welcome home" messages and invitations on the voice mail. We started taking cards out of the bags to share with Emily, but she could handle only a few before she wanted to stop. I could see the wisdom of Kari's insight that Emily might need to let the world in gradually.

The next day Emily was moody and uncharacteristically shy because she couldn't walk and had to be in a wheelchair to go any real distances. This was embarrassing to her and she was self-conscious about the way she looked. She had not yet lost her hair from chemotherapy, but her face was swollen from the steroids and she was retaining so much water that her clothes didn't fit her well. She had to sleep in one of Kari's shirts. Everything about her body was uncomfortable.

We got her a child-sized walker and I put tennis balls on the feet to make it easier to push along the floor, but it was still a lot of effort to get her to take a few steps. Her legs were sore and her muscles were weak, so walking was not pleasant. I cheered her on, but cheering didn't rouse her much. Then I made the mistake of bribing her, offering her a trip to the ice cream shop if she walked across the room. From then on, we had protracted negotiations each time I wanted her to get up to her feet. We had to get a new coloring book, or paints or markers. She won many of these negotiations and I remember saying, "You could be a lawyer with those negotiation skills!"

———•◦•———

Once we adjusted to being back home, we made an appointment to meet Dr. Jim Powell, a pediatric oncologist who had worked at Hershey but now worked at Mount Nittany Medical Center. He managed the pediatric oncology patients who were being treated at Hershey but lived locally, so that they didn't have to make that two-hour drive as often. He was a very nice man, a family man with an amazing wife, Miriam, and two adorable sons. We had an instant connection with him. Mount Nittany Medical Center is only a twenty-five-minute drive from home, and Dr. Powell agreed that we could schedule some of Emily's clinic visits with him. We could call him when Emily had a fever and he could administer antibiotics. He knew Emily's doctors at Hershey, and, with his guidance and care, he promised he'd arrange for Emily to be the first pediatric patient to receive chemo at Mount Nittany. What a relief to have a great doctor so close to home.

———————— ··•●•·· ————————

At our visit with Dr. Powell, he encouraged us to get Emily walking to strengthen her leg muscles, and I thought taking her to our family camp might help. Camp was a rocky mile-long drive down a dirt road through the woods to a clearing near a creek. During hunting season, the men of my father's and grandfather's generation brought their sons to camp every weekend, and those weekends were governed by well-established rules. As a young boy, I watched my older brother Jim go off with Dad when he turned five, and I could hardly wait to be old enough to join them. My grandfather's generation were World War II veterans, and they liked a rugged atmosphere. They fed us buckwheat pancakes for breakfast and C rations for lunch and dinner. You had to be twelve years old before they let you handle a gun, so for those first seven years what you really were learning was how to be a man.

Every morning the men divided into two groups, with half the men (and boys) up in the hunting stands and the other half working as pushers. The pushers formed a line and walked through the forest, flushing the game in front of them as they advanced toward the hunting stands. As a young boy, I'd be alongside either my dad or his uncles (who were close in age to him) as we strode strongly forward, making as much noise as we could. That was so different from up in the hunting stands, when we had to be quiet.

The job of the young kids in the stands was to use the binoculars to spot deer or bears. Most of the time, though, we were silent and alert to any twitch of a branch or footfall on the forest floor. I remember how hard it was to sit very still. Also, I remember being in awe of my dad, Big Jim, who was six feet and broad in the shoulders. I always thought he was one of the strongest men in Philipsburg. He was the dad who, when a fight broke out at a party, waded into the crush of people and separated the combatants. When Big Jim laid his big mitts on you, you felt it, and you straightened up right away. On the walkie-talkies we used to communicate in the forest, his handle was Poppa Bear, and it suited him.

Then my generation took over and the place started to change. My brothers and other members of our family are pretty good cooks, so we worked on upgrading the kitchen and began throwing a big full-week party after Thanksgiving, right around the opening of buck season. Where it used to be lots of trucks and heaps of dirt bikes on the land next to the camp, in our era it became lines of ATVs. Friends and their families come from all over the area, over the back roads and through the streams and down the hillsides, until they get to our place for some brisket. And the other thing that changed was that my brothers and I included our daughters.

We kept the family tradition of stocking the creek with trout in the spring so the kids could learn to fish, but we added in some palomino fish because the colors delighted the little girls and the boys, too. When I started taking Emily up in the hunting stand, I never expected her to want to shoot, although it would have been fine with me if she did. I wanted her to have what I had had with my dad, that quiet time looking around at nature.

I started taking Emily out to camp from the moment she could sit up in a car seat, but never during hunting season, so we could spend time together in the woods. By the time she was three or four, able to walk far enough to check out a porcupine, we'd go out every weekend, just the two of us. Emily loved to climb, so I would let her go first up the long ladder to the hunting stand. I would be right behind her to catch her if she missed a rung. Up there with me she learned to distinguish the different birdsongs, and to look for porcupines, raccoons, and turkeys. She even named pairs of does and their fawns. This was my way of opening this part of my world to her in whatever way she wanted to take it. She loved being there with me. This was why I hoped that getting her to the hunting camp might encourage her to walk.

As we drove slowly down the dirt road to camp, she was scanning the trees for birds and the forest floor for animals. I stopped the SUV next to the camp and got out her wheelchair and her walker, hoping she'd choose to walk, but she did not. I picked her up out of the SUV, gently placed her into the wheelchair, and maneuvered it over a rocky path to the bridge so she could look at the fish and scatter some food for them. Then I pushed the chair over to sit at the side of the stream for a while.

I scanned these familiar hillsides as Emily and I sat silently by the creek. I knew every contour of the hill, every stream, and all the hallows. By the time I was ten and Jim was eleven, we'd saved up to buy dirt bikes. Every chance we got, we were kicking up dust, rocks flying in our wake, as we splashed through the streams to the tops of the strip-mined mountains, heading home only when we saw the sun getting low in the sky. Had my love of this land given Emily leukemia? The doctors said they didn't know what caused her disease. Was it genetics? Did some inherited genetic defect in the body awaken the cancer in someone who was vulnerable to that form of the disease? Could the medicine I had been taking for years for Crohn's disease have somehow caused Emily's leukemia? Or was it mostly environmental? Had my brothers and I splashed through toxins in the streams that ran down the sides of the strip-mined hills? The doctors told us not to focus on what might have caused her cancer because we would never have a definitive answer. They suggested we use all of our energy to focus on getting Emily through this. But I still couldn't stop thinking, *Is this horrible thing that happened to her in some way my fault?*

I kept recalling something that had happened the summer before. I had a powerful bug spray that I kept in my SUV, the kind that had DEET in it, to help me fend off the bloodthirsty ticks that attacked us at camp. Also, that summer, Emily loved an apple-flavored spray candy they sold at the concession stands at the high school softball games. One Saturday when we pulled into our driveway, I had just unstrapped Emily from her booster seat when a friend stopped by. While he and I chatted, Emily pretended to drive for a while, but it wasn't too long before she was on the floor rummaging around underneath the seat and found the bug spray that had fallen out of my bag.

By the time I said goodbye to my friend, I caught her in the foot well with a terrified look on her face. Emily was alarmed by the taste of the "candy" and ran into the house to ask Kari what to do about the candy that was making her mouth burn. That's when we realized she'd sprayed DEET in her mouth. We rushed to the ER, worried that she had swallowed the toxin. The doctor there told me not to worry because it was a small amount, but I worried still as I was sitting by the stream with Emily, trying to find a way to blame myself for the pain that had happened to my blameless little girl.

———— ··●·· ————

At camp, Emily and I sat for a while in the comfortable silence we'd built over the years. There was so much she had learned just by being there with me. I remembered how, the summer before, we had been walking when a family of turkeys, a mom, dad, and their chicks, walked some distance up ahead of us and Emily froze. Then it seemed like the turkeys disappeared. Emily looked upset and a bit confused, as if she had imagined them. I crouched down and told her softly to stay still and have patience, which is very hard for a child that age, but she held her ground. I'll never forget the delight on her face when the ferns and brush started to move, and the turkey family skittered from the underbrush and dashed across the forest floor. No better way to learn the virtue of patience than through such an experience, which gave her such a wonderful reward.

That afternoon at camp I could hear the chickadees, bluebirds, and whip-poor-wills over the rush of the stream in front of us. I saw Emily's eyes searching the wood until she caught sight of a fawn in a beam of sunlight, its graceful head responding to small sounds in the woods around.

"Do you want to take a couple of steps, Emily?"

"No, Daddy. I just want to sit here."

"Just a couple of steps, huh? Might help to get your feet on rough ground to strengthen some of the muscles you don't get to use much indoors."

"No. I'll just sit."

I wanted so much for my girl. I wanted more than she could ever know and maybe ever imagine, but maybe that was too much. I should take her where she was, as Kari always advised, and be happy with what we had, with this moment right now in the forest, where we didn't have to struggle at all.

When she was ready to go home, I pushed her in the wheelchair back to the SUV, picked her up, and strapped her into her booster seat, then stowed the walker and the wheelchair in the back. When we started back up the dirt road the afternoon was cool enough that we didn't need the air conditioner.

I opened the windows to the SUV so we could fill our lungs with that forest smell, the trees and the vegetation turning into mulch on the forest floor. I looked at her in the rearview mirror and saw a little girl who was getting stronger every day. Her eyes were half-closed in blissful contentment, and I felt so grateful to be home.

Chapter 7

I LOVE LUCY

The good news of July was that Emily was in remission! The chemo had worked, and the consolidation treatment phase began. Even with daily chemotherapy pills, she felt pretty good and the nausea was at a minimum. Several times a week a physical therapist came to work with her on walking. She wasn't putting her heels all the way down to the floor, so the physical therapist put squeakers on her heels. Whenever her heel hit the ground it let out a little *eep* so that she knew she'd made it all the way to the floor on that step. She liked the sound so much that she started stomping around the house, which made me and Kari laugh.

We'd take her out for a walk, but she'd want to come home right away. She was trying hard, but her legs still hurt too much for her to go very far. I'd try to get her laughing with some goofy stunt, but some days the most I could get from her was my bare-minimum one smile a day.

As Emily's legs got stronger with her *eep* therapy, she stopped using her walker and said she wanted to go swimming. I knew how much Emily missed swimming in the hot days of summer. She'd gained more than ten pounds from the steroids, and her body was bulky and uncomfortable.

Now that she was off steroids, the weight started to fall off. She was less moody, more herself at home, but swimming would still offer her the mobility she was missing on her feet. It was hard to tell Emily that she couldn't go swimming because her PICC line couldn't get wet. She would have to wait until the doctors swapped out the temporary PICC line for a Mediport.

The surgeon made a one-inch incision in the middle of her chest and inserted the port under her skin. Each time Emily needed chemotherapy a nurse would insert a needle through her skin and into the middle of the implanted port, which was called "accessing the port," and it would deliver the medicine through a catheter, and into her bloodstream. A few days after the port was placed and the insertion wound was healed, Emily was cleared to swim at last, but we had to wait until dusk because chemo made her sensitive skin burn more easily.

At sunset, we drove to Greg's house, where I lowered Emily gently into his pool in her floaty. She held on to me for a while before she kicked away from me, giggling at the joy of moving around in the water. It was a happy time for us, and for that hour of swimming we forgot about needles and chemo and leg infections. We swam and laughed, both of us happy that Emily could do something normal once more.

After that she swam almost every day, which was great therapy because the more she swam, the stronger her legs became. Emily was so proud of how she could do almost everything she used to do, just a little more slowly. The one thing she couldn't do was climb the stairs without holding on to the handrail. The physical therapist spent some part of each session talking to her about the goal of being able to bound up the stairs like a five-year-old in time for the start of kindergarten.

In late summer, Emily was offered the chance to throw out the first pitch for a local minor league baseball team, the State College Spikes, which was holding a cancer fund-raiser. She surprised me by saying yes. We practiced her throw in the backyard, but I still wasn't sure if she'd want to do it when the day came around. She did! She made her way out to the mound without a walker or a wheelchair and took a firm grip on the ball, just like we had practiced. Although her pitch didn't make it all the way to home plate, it was strong and straight, and she got big applause from all her new fans in the stadium.

The organizer of the event, Kim Kawa-Ludwig, called Kari a few days later and said she had a wonderful surprise she wanted to give to Emily: a puppy.

After Emily went to bed that night, Kari and I talked it over. We'd never had a dog in the house because I love them too much to leave them alone all day when we're out at work. But Emily had responded so strongly to Jasper, the therapy dog in the hospital. She still talked about him, and Kari said Emily imagined owning a dog. She'd even named her imaginary dog Lucy. So why not? we decided. Everything in our lives had changed so much in the last two months, why was I holding on to this cranky decision made years ago? Changing my mind might help Emily heal.

The next day Kari and I met with Kim halfway between our houses, in the small town of Osceola Mills, and were introduced to two adorable puppies, a white one and a speckled one. Even such tiny creatures have personalities. The white one had a bit of elegance in the way she threw her head, and she was frisky, eager to engage. The smaller puppy was a calico, with patches of brown and black on her white fur. The smaller pup held back, waiting for Kari to reach out to her.

"Full disclosure," Kim said to Kari. "There might be something amiss in the multicolored one. She got carsick on the ride here."

"Well, then she's the one for us!" said Kari. She took the puppy up close to her face for a snuggle. "Yes, you are the one. This little baby has a lot in common with Emily."

Kari wanted to give Emily the dog immediately, but I'm all for the big reveal. We'd already invited some of the family over for a barbecue that Saturday, so we decided to invite a few more. We knew everyone would want to witness this.

But what would we do with the puppy for the next two days? Kari said I should leave her with my folks, and I laughed at the thought of this wisp of a creature in the hands of Big Jim. When we were kids, my brothers and I always knew that people wouldn't mess with us because they knew Big Jim would come looking for them if they did. In the last decade Big Jim had had to slow down. His strength, ironically, had created his weakness. He'd fallen out of the bucket one day when he was working on a transformer and broken his back. Being Big Jim, he shook off the pain and never went to a doctor. The next time he fell, a year later, he did serious damage to that poorly healed injury and had to retire on a disability pension. While he tended to his broken back, his roughness receded, and he transformed from Big Jim to Poppa Bear. The tender, generous, and loving parts of his big heart moved to the foreground. He was more sentimental and cried easily (and was embarrassed about that), but that solid love of his family always came through.

I walked into my parents' house with the itty-bitty carrier that contained the puppy and rested it on the table next to my dad.

"What's this, now?" he said gruffly.

I opened the gate to the carrier and brought out the puppy nestled in a fluffy pink blanket. My dad leaned forward to get a look.

"Aw!" he said. "Aw!"

"We got Emily a puppy. We're going to give it to her Saturday at the barbecue. Could you keep her here until then?"

"Oh, sure, sure," he said. "How could you not love that cutie?"

Dad placed the tiny puppy in the palm of his great big mitt and brought her closer to his face. They took a good look at each other.

"Aw!" he said again. "You know, Tom, anytime you don't want her to be alone, just say the word. She's always welcome here."

———··●··———

We had to work hard to hide the preparations for the party. Emily knew we were having a backyard barbecue, but she had no idea how large it was going to be.

Before the party, we sent Emily out with my mom. When they returned, Emily was shocked by all the familiar cars parked in front of the house. Mom and Emily came up around the house and into the garden, and Emily came straight over to me and Kari. The crowd was silent, all eyes following Emily as she made her way across the yard.

"Emily, you've been so good and so brave these last months we wanted to give you something special," Kari said.

Kari reached into the dog carrier and gently took out a blanket with the dog snuggled within.

Kari bent down to offer Emily the little bundle. Emily gasped.

"Lucy!" she said softly.

It was the whisper heard by everyone there. No one dared applaud the delicacy of this moment, but nearly everyone uttered, "Aw!"

Watching Emily stare at Lucy was like standing in sunshine. For Emily, there was no other world than Lucy. That summer we had a new swing set on the other side of the yard from the one I'd built for Emily, a light tan one with benches and a roof to offer some shade. We brought Emily and Lucy to the bench swing that Kari had made cozy with pillows as she had anticipated Emily's need for privacy. Nestled there together, Emily and Lucy got to know each other. As people left, they'd visit the swing on their way out to bid their goodbyes.

Emily had been sleeping with us since she came home from the hospital because it was just easier. If we needed to take her temperature or her legs were hurting, we were right there. When Lucy arrived, Emily didn't want to sleep in our bed anymore. She wanted to be alone with Lucy.

Emily was very interested in the routine of caring for a puppy. She asked all sorts of questions about what was going to happen to Lucy at the vet's office because she had a lot of experience with doctors. She also asked the vet about feeding Lucy and exercise. The doctor gave her a chart to fill out when she weighed Lucy each week. She even trained Lucy how to step on the scale. Lucy was always up to something, chewing strings, buttons, toes, Polly Pocket shoes—almost anything she found on the floor. Emily was always prying Lucy's mouth open to rescue what she had stashed inside.

We all love Lucy! Emily still carries her around like a baby and Lucy is just fine with that because she likes to be held and cuddled. When we first got her she was a little hesitant and scared, but now she loves to explore and play. She chews EVERYTHING. Her favorite thing to chew on is toes, which Emily thinks is pretty funny. Lucy also goes crazy when she hears newspaper being crinkled, which makes Emily giggle really hard. Emily couldn't wait to tell all the nurses and doctors that she has a new puppy. It's been wonderful for her and also good for us...gives us all something else to focus on!

—Kari's journal
August 12, 2010

Emily was excited about starting kindergarten, so Kari and I hadn't told her we weren't sure whether this was a good idea. If she started, she was sure to miss a lot of class, but since she was already reading, we didn't think she would fall behind. We were more concerned about all the germs she'd be exposed to when she was surrounded by other kids. Plus being out on her own took a lot of energy, and we weren't sure she had enough to last the whole day at school. We decided that trying to make life as normal as possible for her was the best decision.

We worked with the school nurse to ensure that Emily could come in to have her temperature taken at the nurse's office each day at lunch. We talked to her kindergarten teacher about keeping an eye on Emily in case she started to look tired or unfocused in class, because it might be a sign that she was getting sick. Once we were feeling more confident about the great support she was going to receive at school, we talked to Emily about using hand sanitizer, washing her hands, and doing what she could not to catch any stray colds that might be moving through the children in her kindergarten class.

A few weeks before school started, I took Emily to camp one day with Lucy beside her in the backseat. Lucy was very excited to be going to camp, racing all over the seat to look out the windows, and Emily was laughing at how animated Lucy was.

When we got to camp, Emily was eager to get out of the SUV, following Lucy. I brought out the wheelchair, but Emily was already taking steps. She was slow, but she was walking. They walked down to the edge of the creek. I brought out the fishing gear and set us up to fish. Lucy raced back and forth for a while, but soon she calmed down as we cast our lines, reeled them back, and talked about school starting and getting into a regular routine.

When we were done fishing, I helped Emily back into the SUV. This day was pretty close to the way we spent time before Emily got sick. We cranked the windows down to get fresh air and I looked at Emily in the back, Lucy nestled in her lap and her eyes closed, enjoying the warmth of Lucy and the breeze. As we picked up speed on the main road, I saw some strands of her hair—just a few—swooshing away out the window and into the summer air.

Chapter 8

THON

It looks like Emily is going to lose her hair after all. She's lost about half of what she had just over the last few days and there is hair everywhere! When she wakes up in the morning the pillow is covered and when you run a brush through it, it just comes out in clumps. She doesn't seem upset by it at all and even laughs when she sees how much is coming out. She's collecting it in a baggy, which she actually thinks is kind of fun. The side of her head is pretty much bald but the top is still long enough to cover the sides (almost looks like a long mohawk!) so as long as we comb her hair straight down it still covers most of the bald spots but it looks very thin.

—Kari's journal
October 24, 2010

That moment when I saw Emily's hair flying out the window as we drove home from camp I worried that Emily would be upset, but she surprised us. Sometimes the short hairs of her pixie cut would fall onto her arms or clothes and she'd laugh as she flicked it away. It was the same when Kari brushed her hair and the brush was thick with strands she'd pulled easily from Emily's scalp. Emily didn't seem to mind. Kari was the one who was the most upset by it. What would her hair be like when it came back?

Maybe Emily had spent all that emotion when she got so mad that we gave her a haircut that first weekend she was in the hospital. And it also might have been my campaign of saying as often as possible, "Hair doesn't matter. It will always grow back." She still had most of her hair the day she started kindergarten.

The day Emily first took the bus ride to kindergarten ranks up there with the day we got married and the day of Emily's birth as one of those days I will never forget. She was so excited the night before, I didn't think she'd go to sleep. We told her good students need a full eight hours so their minds absorb all the knowledge that the teacher is trying to offer. This got her into bed, but before we turned off the light, she told us she knew the first day would just be a lot of games so she didn't really need eight hours. Well, she did, I said as I laid Lucy across Emily's feet, the sure sign that it was time for her to go off to dreamland.

They were both still sound asleep when Kari got Lucy to wake Emily up that next morning. Kari stood Lucy so she was facing Emily from the foot of the bed, and Lucy barked and jumped back and forth, ready to play. But Emily was all business that morning. We'd packed Emily's backpack the night before. Kari made her a big breakfast of scrambled eggs and oatmeal. We wanted to walk her to the bus, but she refused. She insisted on walking down our front steps herself and making her own way to the school bus, waving to us from the window as it pulled away.

We thought about her often throughout the day as we waited for the bus to bring her back and for Lucy to leap out of my arms to greet Emily, a little bundle of wiggles at her feet. Emily returned from school with a good report. Her teacher was the greatest and she already had made two friends.

With Emily at school and me and Kari back to work, we had a sense of life returning to normal, but that sense was fragile. Emily still had weekly daylong appointments at Hershey that might or might not end up with her being admitted for observation, and we never knew when Emily's temperature would reach 100.5 degrees and we'd be on our way to the Mount Nittany ER and perhaps on from there to Hershey.

I used to keep a close eye on the Nittany Lions football schedule because Emily seemed to spike a fever almost every time Penn State, the university near the Mount Nittany Medical Center, had a home football game. I dreaded that journey to the ER on those days. The nurses could barely hear me describe what was wrong with Emily over the ruckus of the injured or intoxicated football fans, and we usually had to wait for hours for Emily to get treated.

We quickly got leaving for the ER down to a drill. As soon as Emily spiked a fever, I'd call Dad, and my parents would come to get Lucy, usually before we'd made our way out the door. Our duffel bags were always packed, resting in the garage near the SUV. Kari had a bag of crafts and books at the ready, too. And in Emily's bag she had her prayer cloths. Emily clung to those. She'd lay prayer cloths over her head when she had a migraine, and sometimes when she just wanted to tune everything out. When the nurses tried to remove them, Emily would tell them, "No one touches my prayer cloths."

We'd fight our way through the Saturday night chaos until we got her admitted to one of the triage rooms. The doctor would order antibiotics, which would take a few hours to administer. While Emily was on the IV antibiotics, they monitored how she responded. All the time the question hung in the air: Was she sick enough to transfer to Hershey or could they send her home? Usually, she was transferred by ambulance to Hershey to be admitted for a few days.

The waiting was unbearable for all of us, hours crammed into those small, curtained-off ER spaces. I remember once waking up on the floor next to Emily's bed as a nurse stepped over me to check on her. I'd come into the room and found Kari asleep in the chair, Emily resting in the bed, and no place for me to lay my head. I was so tired I decided I'd just lie down on the floor. My back was stiff and cramping and I had a terrible headache the next morning.

A few times Emily was transported to Hershey in an ambulance. I remember one chaotic ambulance ride where we must have had a rookie crew of EMTs. Kari was inside with Emily and I was following behind in our car when I saw the driver swerving so badly that she ran a car in the adjacent lane off the road. I called Kari to see what was going on, but she didn't have time to answer. She was dealing with a crisis of her own. As she sat there tending to Emily, she came to recognize that the EMT was blowing her nose and coughing a wet cough, and it was escalating quickly. Kari was spending all her attention trying to shield Emily from the germs.

Our weekly visits to Hershey's outpatient oncology clinic began before sunrise, when we left Philipsburg for the two-hour drive. As soon as we got to the clinic, we all donned surgical masks to protect the children from picking up germs from us and from each other. The nurses put numbing cream on the children's chests so that accessing the Mediports were less painful, and together the families waited for an hour or more for the cream to take effect.

With the stress all of us were under, this was a part of the appointment we appreciated. While the child life specialists played games and did crafts with the children, the parents chatted, updating each other on their child's condition, and sharing our worries with the only people in the world who truly understood how we felt. In the waiting room our hearts were open to each other. When a new family arrived, the group embraced them. If we saw a parent sitting alone, one of the parents would sit next to that mom, maybe place an arm around her shoulder, waiting to see if she wanted to talk. The children knew to welcome other children, too. The first day Emily arrived, a girl named Bella, who also had leukemia, explained to her how much getting her port accessed was going to hurt, but that she would get used to it. Weeks later, Emily was the one who was giving this same advice to the newcomers.

When Emily's name was called, our anxiety about what was going to happen with her Mediport began. After each time the nurses accessed the port, they protected it with a thin, sticky plastic film called Tegaderm that adhered strongly to the skin. Ripping the Tegaderm off was agony for Emily. When we got to the examination room, Emily sat in my lap so I could hold her arms as the nurse ripped away the bandage. Then the nurse would swab the area with alcohol and access the port. Each time Emily screamed in pain, but she was also afraid. She knew this was just the beginning of being poked and prodded.

Next came the blood draw. Sometimes the nurses collected five or six tubes of blood. Usually she had a lumbar puncture followed by chemotherapy injected into her spinal fluid to make sure cancer cells didn't grow there. This was followed by a bone marrow aspiration to check for cancer cells in her bone marrow and make sure she was still in remission. After a visit with Dr. Ungar, Emily would receive IV chemotherapy that she knew would make her sick later that day and maybe the next.

We'd take our place at the chemo infusion center, each family separated from the others by curtains. The nurse connected bags of chemotherapy and fluids from Emily's port to the IV pump. Sometimes the IV infusions took thirty minutes, but sometimes they took up to eight hours.

As we watched the medicine drip slowly into Emily, sometimes we heard children crying or throwing up at the other chemo stations. Often when we heard the soft sobs of the other overwhelmed parents, I'd leave Emily's side and go to comfort them and often we got the same in return. This reassurance usually came without words. A simple hug and a kind gaze were all that was needed to show other parents that we knew what they were going through and that we were in this together.

During the chemo infusion, we anxiously awaited the blood work results. If her red blood cells or platelets were low, then she would have to stay at clinic longer to get a blood or platelet transfusion. If Emily's white blood cell count was low, it meant her immune system was weak, and she would have to miss school for a few days to avoid germs. So much hung on these visits, yet nurses and child life specialists managed to keep the atmosphere light. There was always laughter and jokes.

After the procedures and infusions were done, we often drove to Friendly's across the street from the medical center for a quick bite to eat or an ice cream treat before heading home. We knew that at some point during the drive Emily would have to use the restroom, so we usually stopped at the Harley-Davidson dealership about an hour and a half from the hospital. I often ended up buying something, a T-shirt or a little motorcycle toy; because we were such regular customers of their facilities, I thought we should pay them back a little. We might have to deal with Emily being sick on the drive home, which was miserable for her, because the last place you want to be when you are nauseous is riding in a car for a long period. Sometimes she would be fine, and we would roll the windows down and sing. It just depended on the type of chemo she'd gotten and how her body responded. We came home exhausted, knowing we had to do it all again the next week.

In October, when we took Emily to Hershey for her weekly chemo treatment, the doctor became concerned about her legs again. Her right calf was swollen and red. They decided to admit her so that they could give her IV antibiotics and keep an eye on the redness and swelling.

Emily perked up when she heard that she was being admitted because she was excited to return to the playroom, and she was already boasting about how she was going to beat me at air hockey because she wasn't in a wheelchair anymore. When Kari mentioned she was disappointed that Emily would miss Halloween, the nurse told her she wouldn't miss it at all. The hospital had plenty of costumes for her to choose from, and all the young patients were going trick-or-treating around the hospital the next day.

That next morning when Emily sat up to eat, she noticed that she'd left a bunch of hair behind on the pillow. I could see the alarmed look on Kari's face, but before Emily could even react, I repeated, "Hair doesn't matter. It will always grow back." Then I saw that twinkle Emily gets in her eyes right before she's going to challenge me.

"If hair doesn't matter," Emily said, "then we can cut off all of yours."

I paused for a second. She'd caught me in my hypocrisy. I meant her hair didn't matter, not mine. So I grabbed the electric razor from my duffel bag and popped out the beard-trimmer attachment to hand to Emily.

"Okay," I said. "You shave my head and then I'll shave yours."

I laid my head on her lap and she went to work. To be honest with you, I thought there was no way that small clipper manipulated by her little hand would give me much of a pruning. When I pulled myself up and took a look in the mirror, I had just a thin layer of fuzz. It was shocking to see.

"My turn to shave yours!" I said. And I did.

When I was done, we were completely bald. I took her over to the mirror so she could get a look at the two of us together. I saw a look, a mood, come over her face. It was not shock or anger, but gratitude. Emily put her little arms around my neck and gave me a kiss on the cheek.

"I love you, Daddy," she said.

———————··•●•··———————

The next day, we had a visit from Penn State students who participate in THON.

The Penn State Dance Marathon, or THON, is a forty-six-hour dance marathon that the students hold every year on the third weekend in February. The event raises money to financially support the pediatric cancer families who are treated at Hershey Medical Center. Nearly 15,000 Penn State students participate in THON each year. THON has supported thousands of families, and now we were among them. We were grateful for that monetary support, but on this day in October we learned how much more support those students had to offer. Each child and family are adopted by a Penn State student organization, and our family was adopted by the university's public relations student society, the PRSSA.

We were in Emily's room watching Nickelodeon when we heard a commotion in the hallway, the sound of high voices and laughter that always precede a visit from THON. The nursing staff lets families know when the THON kids are coming because not every family is ready for the energy of a half dozen excitable young people. We were eager, though, and when the blast of joy of their arrival reached our ears, Emily asked us to turn off the television. Then there they were, decked out in their Penn State Nittany Lions gear, framed by the six window panes in the door to Emily's room. I saw Ariana, the junior who a few weeks earlier had shepherded us around the THON Harvest Festival, walking us between the corn maze and the pumpkin patch. We all liked Ariana, a native of Pittston, a small town in the northeastern part of Pennsylvania, close to Scranton. We were hoping she'd be one of the students allowed into Emily's room, but two of the other students came inside to visit instead.

I went into the hallway to thank Ariana and the others for coming, and Emily insisted she wanted to give them all Silly Bandz, these colorful, stretchy wristbands she'd been collecting from the doctors and the nurses on the unit.

Later that day one of the students who had visited Emily's room, Becky Salman, wrote a note for us on the CaringBridge blog that really touched Kari and me. Becky wrote that she loved and admired our family, even from that brief visit. Many in her family had survived cancer, and she wrote that she didn't know which was harder: to have cancer or "to watch it happen to someone you would give your life for.…When all is in the past Emily will have her strength, her wonderful parents by her side, and a story she will share with others who are in the shoes she is in now. She will be a role model and will inspire others with her bravery and experiences."

What we loved about that note from Becky was her positive attitude that matched our own, and her powerful heartfelt message. She wrote that she followed Kari's blog and that "Emily is in my every prayer. The little angel has not left my mind since I had the opportunity to meet her on Tuesday. Thank you for letting us be a part of your child's life." When we got out of the hospital and back to Philipsburg, we invited Becky to come visit. We had no idea what a big part of our lives she was about to become.

From the moment she arrived in our home, Becky fit right in with our family. She was excitable and flamboyant, a force of nature, and all of that came through as joy. Many times, when people came to visit Emily, Kari and I acted as entertainment coordinators, trying to think of something to do that Emily and the visitors could both enjoy. Becky came ready to play, with a satchel full of Silly String and prepared to become a dog or a space alien, or whatever kind of character would make Emily laugh. She walked in the door and straight off to Emily's room, like her kindergarten friends did. We heard them giggling and goofing around until they were ready to eat. All of us agreed that Becky was welcome anytime she wanted to visit.

In November, when Emily returned to school after a hospital stay, she was wearing a hat to cover her bald head and felt a little self-conscious about it. When she entered her kindergarten class, she saw that all her classmates and teachers were wearing hats, too. The principal had allowed the students to show their support for her if they wanted to do so, and many of them did, building on the wave of support we received from all our neighbors in Philipsburg.

Right before Thanksgiving, we were sitting at the kitchen table going over the mountain of expenses we faced, not knowing how we were going to come up with the money to pay the bills not covered by insurance. We were looking at a $1,000 bill for an ambulance ride to Mount Nittany Medical Center. Then the doorbell rang, and I went to answer.

"Tom Whitehead?" the visitor asked.

"Yes, that's me," I said.

"You don't know me, but everyone at my church has been following along on your family's blog, and we all pray every week for Emily," he said.

"Thank you," I said. "Thank you from all of us. We feel every prayer. And when it's hard for us, we think of all of you pulling for us, even people we don't know, and we're grateful."

"We had a fund-raiser for you," he said. "It's not much, but it's something."

I took the envelope from the stranger and then I took his hand. "Tell everyone at your church how grateful we are to you. Please keep Emily in your prayers."

"You know we will," he said.

I took the envelope back to the kitchen table and laid the money out between me and Kari: ten one-hundred-dollar bills, exactly what we needed to pay for the ambulance.

"There's something to this," I said to Kari with a grin.

From this, of course, I took hope. How could we fail with so much goodwill and generosity on our side?

From this Kari took urgency. "We don't know what's coming, Tom," she said. "We have to live right now, every minute. We need to show Emily as much of the world as we can."

"I think we're doing okay."

"Every child should see New York City at Christmas."

"New York City! I hate big cities."

"You've never been there," Kari said. "How do you know?"

"I don't have to go there to know. From everything I've heard, I wouldn't like it and it wouldn't like me."

"This is not for you; it's for Emily," Kari said, and that was a fair point.

"OK," I agreed. "Let's make a plan to go."

Just before New Year's Day, we headed out of Philipsburg toward New York City and the Algonquin Hotel on West Forty-Fourth Street. I was dreading it. I didn't want to fight our way through those dense streets, past the hard-faced buildings, through the rude and noisy crowds. For Kari and Emily to have a beautiful visit, I would have to keep this attitude to myself. Little did I know how quickly the people of the City of New York would change my mind.

Becky's family lives right outside New York City in New Jersey, and when she heard we were making our maiden voyage east, she insisted that we stop by to meet her parents, Michael and Natasha. I was especially interested in meeting Becky's so-called Soviet father. Becky's family had emigrated from Russia in the 1980s with only a suitcase and $200, and from that built their American dream. Her dad had made a good living in real estate and her mom worked behind the Red Door at the Elizabeth Arden salon in Manhattan. All this American prosperity had not changed Michael's Russian-style fatherhood.

The stories Becky told of tangling with her father were hilarious. When Michael bought Becky a car, he was upset that she was playing the radio so loud she would not be able to hear honks or emergency vehicles coming up behind her. And while she promised him she'd turn the volume down, he could still hear her coming down the street. One day Becky jumped into the car and jabbed at the radio to find her father had removed it. She was furious! She still was mad at her dad when she told that story.

There was a reason Becky and Emily were friends, despite their age difference. Neither one like to be told no. They both liked to be in charge. When Becky told these stories, I saw Emily and me when she got to high school. I could see a touch of Becky in Emily's defiance and her smarts.

The next morning, when we pulled up in front of the Algonquin, a crew of porters swarmed around the SUV and unloaded all our bags. As we walked to the front desk to check in, Emily spied Matilda, the hotel's resident cat, laid out like a queen on her chaise lounge. Matilda sure ruled the lobby from there. She was plump from all the treats she received from everyone who passed by. Her body was grayish white with darker-gray fur on her face and legs and snow-white paws. Emily crouched to pet Matilda on the head, grinning as the cat swiveled her head around to receive Emily's touch. What a great beginning to our visit. Every time we passed through the hotel Emily was looking to see what Matilda was up to.

We were really stretching our money to take this trip, which meant our room was small, a big motivation to get us out into the street. Becky met us at the hotel, a bit worried about how this family of country bumpkins would handle life in the big city. It had snowed heavily the night before we arrived, and the city workers had piled the snow high at the edge of the sidewalk.

Kari had bundled Emily up carefully in multiple layers. She looked snug in the wheelchair we had borrowed for the trip because Emily's legs were still weak and she had a hard time walking very far. From the moment we turned east on Forty-Fourth Street I felt all my negative opinions about New York City start to slip away. We didn't have to fight our way through the streets. The crowds gently parted before Emily's wheelchair and closed back up behind us as soon as we passed. Every time we came to a corner, hands reached out from the crowd to help lift Emily's wheelchair safely onto the sidewalk and, before I could thank their owners, those hands disappeared into the mass of strangers supporting us wherever we went.

I wasn't the only person being pushed outside of my comfort zone to give Emily this gift. I kept an eye on Kari, who is anxious in crowds, as we walked toward Rockefeller Plaza to the American Girl doll store. The store was so crowded you could barely move. Emily had received a bald American Girl doll for Christmas, so she was not interested in the store's salon where dolls could get their hair done, but she was interested in the doll hospital. She was also interested in getting her ears pierced there, but it turned out they pierced only the ears of the dolls. I wasn't interested in any of it. This had to be a mother-daughter moment. The noise, the crowds, the colors—it was all too much for me and for Becky. She and I ended up standing outside, tending to Emily's wheelchair. Becky was such a great tour guide for us, taking us to Times Square and over to Toys"R"Us so Emily could ride the Ferris wheel that dominated the center of the store. I don't know how we would have braved it all without her.

We ate a lot of pizza in our room to save money, but I promised that on the last night we were there we'd have a special dinner in the Algonquin dining room. Kari and Emily dressed up for our special meal. We sat in a big red leatherette banquette, served by the greatest waiters, silent and swift in answering our needs before we even mentioned them. Before we ate, Emily insisted on counting out her pills, all seventeen of them. My brilliant girl wanted to get control of all of the aspects of her disease because she'd caught the nurses and the doctors making mistakes. She knew the names of each of her medicines and what they were supposed to do for her, announcing that as she counted them out.

I was so proud of her I guess I didn't realize how sick Emily might look to a stranger. She looked healthy, happy, and beautiful to me. When I asked for the bill the waiter told us that a man on the other side of the restaurant had picked up the check. I didn't get a chance to thank him. He left before we knew his good deed. You'll never again hear a negative word from me about New York City.

In February, Emily was admitted to the hospital for a fever just a few days before THON weekend. She had been looking forward to the weekend for months, and she was extremely anxious to get well so she would not miss it. Even though we were miles away, we were drawn into the action because of the wonderful tradition THON has to kick off the dancing. The children on the cancer unit at Hershey write letters thanking the dancers for what they are about to do. We all wrote letters to the dancers and placed them in the satchel that would be conveyed over land to THON, one hundred miles away, with runners taking three-mile segments. The relay was perfectly timed so that the last runner arrived in the stadium to deliver the letters shortly before the forty-six hours of dancing commenced. We felt so lucky Emily was discharged in time for us to participate in both ends of this great tradition, to write the letters and then to be there when the dancers received them. We celebrated when THON raised close to $10 million. And we were honored to be just a small part of that.

Chapter 9

RELAPSE

As spring arrived, Emily was granted a Make-A-Wish trip to Disney World. When she was first diagnosed, the Make-A-Wish Foundation had approached us about fulfilling whatever wish she had, and we had a tough time deciding what that would be. We even polled the readers of Kari's blog, where the winning choice turned out to be the right one: a trip to Give Kids The World Village near Orlando.

This was much more than just the trip to Disney World that we had imagined. The eighty-four-acre Give Kids The World private village is "right out of a fairy tale," as Kari wrote in her blog. The families who bring their children to the village get to stay free in a community that is designed to fulfill every whim that these kids have. The 600 volunteers make sure that the families want for nothing, and that was clear from the first time we walked out of registration to find our villa. As we tugged our suitcases behind us, an elderly couple in a golf cart pulled up alongside us to offer us lemonade and cookies and to bring us to our rooms. The whole week we were there, we never had to walk if we didn't want to, as there was always a golf cart and drivers standing by or patrolling the lanes.

We ate our meals at the Gingerbread House, where they encouraged us just to stand up from the table and leave the cleanup to them. The Park of Dreams had a heated pool where children ran through spurting fountains, and after that they could take as many pony rides and turns around the carousel as they wanted and eat as much ice cream as they craved. Mickey and Minnie Mouse and the rest of the Disney characters came to the village to visit the kids instead of the other way around.

Honestly, it was hard to believe how great it was, a place where it was Christmas every day—literally, with a present for Emily delivered to the door every morning and a Christmas parade on Thursday complete with snow and a visit from Santa. We were surrounded by gravely ill children, but most of them didn't seem sick at all that week, and Emily was amazingly healthy, too. She was full of energy and eager to do all the fun activities, like play with others on the life-sized Candy Land game. For Kari and me, the most moving part was walking through the Castle of Miracles, a cottage next to a carousel whose ceiling is decorated with tens of thousands of gold stars, each with the name of a child who has visited the village. I especially loved that place, as we were feeling like we were in the middle of a miracle. Emily was doing so great. We felt her getting strong and healthy. Sure, we had our trips to the ER when she spiked a fever, and our many appointments for the chemo and the assessments of how she was doing fighting back the leukemia, but everything was on track for her to be one of the 90 percent of children who beat this terrible disease.

That spring we became closer to Becky and Ariana, the two Penn State students from THON. We had kept asking Becky about Ariana, the PRSSA chair who had charmed us all, especially Emily, when she had showed us around the Harvest Festival the previous fall. Maybe Becky could bring her along on one of her visits? But Becky refused.

She was intimidated by Ariana, who was high up in the THON hierarchy and very serious and studious, the opposite of Becky—or so Becky thought.

We'd learned from the brief encounters we'd had with Ariana over the past few months that she was focused and determined; she'd decided that she would do Penn State's four-year curriculum in just three years. I asked her why she carried with her a huge backpack filled with books everywhere she went. She said this was so she could study whenever she had a spare moment. Kari and I thought she was a great role model for Emily for that reason, and also because of her focus on doing her best and being a leader. If she joined a club, her goal was to be its president. We thought Emily could learn a lot from Ariana.

That spring semester, it turned out that Becky and Ariana were enrolled in a class together, so I nudged Becky to at least have a chat with Ariana. Becky told us there was no way that the two of them would get along. Ariana was the kind of person who thrived by following rules and working her way up the THON hierarchy, Becky surmised. Becky didn't care about rules and lines of authority. I could see it through Becky's eyes: Becky does what she thinks is right and Ariana does what she knows is correct. Becky was sure if they got to know each other they would be enemies, not friends.

One day Becky was late to class and the only seat free was next to Ariana. She stood at the edge of the class, for a moment thinking she'd just split, but she didn't. She took the seat next to Ariana, hoping to bolt the minute class was over. Instead, when class ended, they struck up a conversation about Emily, and they kept talking as they made their way to the Penn State student center called the HUB, and through dinner. They are still talking to this day. At the end of this first marathon conversation, they agreed to visit Emily together.

Kari and I were delighted when Becky said she was bringing Ariana. I was in charge of hope, yes, but I needed help to bring more joy to Emily, and here it was. It was as if we now had three daughters, and Emily had two big sisters, each one very different. All of us, I think, were astonished by the genuine friendship that developed so quickly between two college girls and our five-year-old daughter.

Ariana said she saw Emily as a peer because Emily asked her such mature questions. The second time Becky and Ariana came to visit, Emily asked Ariana why she worked so hard at school. Was it pressure from her parents? Ariana was dumbstruck for a moment. She'd never asked herself that question. "No, it's not my parents," Ariana responded. "It's me."

I wanted Emily to take in Ariana's strong drive to succeed, her pledge that if she was going to be involved in something, she wanted to do her best, to be a leader. From Becky I wanted her to take in the qualities of enthusiasm and generosity. And from both of them, I wanted Emily to learn empathy.

The other part of this friendship was goofiness, like I had with Emily. Emily and Ariana often teamed up against Becky. One time, Emily and Ariana were pretending to be cats and Emily made Becky pretend to be a dog. Becky wanted to be a cat, too, so Emily told her that she could be a cat only if she ate an actual dog treat. Not only did Becky have to eat the treat, but she also had to eat it dipped into her least favorite food, peanut butter. To our surprise, Becky agreed, and I don't think we've ever seen Emily giggle so hard.

When Easter came along, my mom invited the girls to join our celebration. Ariana was going home for the holiday, but Becky, who is Jewish, had never been to an Easter celebration before and was really excited to come. I'll never forget me and Emily going to pick up Becky at her apartment at State College. Becky was carrying an oversized Easter basket. As she approached the car, the wind kicked up and we laughed till our sides hurt as we watched her chasing colorful plastic eggs and fake grass around the parking lot. She would just get a few back into the basket when the wind would toss them out onto the pavement again. Becky looked so elegant in her pastel Easter outfit, but she was swearing like a sailor as she chased those eggs and grass around the parking lot, unaware that Emily and I were sitting in the SUV, watching her struggle.

It was no shock at all that, as Emily's birthday approached, she instructed Kari and me that she really needed us to plan three birthday parties: one for her elementary school friends, one for the family, and one for her college friends, so that's what we did. Her birthday is early enough in May that the college kids were still in town. I rented a bus that could hold twenty-five and drove it over to Penn State to pick up her guests, but more than that showed up at the party. I enlisted Pappy Rob, who is an incredible cook, to tend to the grill, making hot dogs, burgers, and his delicious grilled chicken. The grandmas were more than generous, adding side dishes to the ones Kari made. I rented a large bouncy house—eighteen feet square and fourteen feet high—and dumped a whole bottle of dish soap on its floor. When I turned on the hose inside of it, the college kids were slipping all over the place and laughing.

It was such a happy beginning to the summer, to Emily's sixth year. We'd beaten leukemia, or so it seemed. It had been tough, but the chemotherapy was working. People started complaining on the blog that Kari wasn't posting enough. She didn't have much to say because weeks went by without complications, requiring only routine clinic visits. When Emily started first grade, we felt like we had emerged from a dark tunnel.

Emily began first grade last week! She was not happy about going back. The first day she went to the school nurse in the first two hours...once because her hand hurt and the second time because her belly hurt. She ended up staying all day but I asked her why she wanted to come home and she replied, "Because I already know everything and I was bored." The past few days have been better though, and she actually has been learning new things that she finds interesting...such as the lifecycle of the butterfly. I said to her "so you ARE learning new things at school" and then she just rolled her eyes at me. She's very picky about what she wears and anything I try putting in her hair is imme-diately pulled out (barrettes, hairbands, etc.). Apparently those things are not "in" right now and "none of the girls wear things in their hair."

—Kari's journal
September 8, 2011

Our lives seemed more like the lives of other families now. Emily was complaining about the things that other little girls complain about, like what she was wearing and how boring school could be. When we went to Vancouver in September for my union convention, we didn't feel we had much to worry about, although I was fortunate enough to be seated next to an executive from the Vancouver Children's Hospital on the plane and got his contact number, and the name of a pediatric oncologist there, just in case our confidence was misplaced.

We stayed in a beautiful hotel in the center of town, the Fairmont, which, like the Algonquin, had resident pets: two dogs. Emily loved play-ing with them. We couldn't help but compare her energy and joy on this trip with her quiet demeanor when we'd been in New York for Christmas in 2010. Instead of being in a wheelchair, she ran through the lobby to see the dogs under her own power.

When we got a day free to see the sights, we visited the park to walk across the Capilano Suspension Bridge. This bridge is 230 feet above a river and trees and 430 feet long. I'm used to being up high in the bucket, so looking down at this dizzying sight didn't rattle me, nor did it rattle Emily. She literally skipped across the bridge, stopping only to help a woman who was overcome with fear at the midpoint. Emily was so kind. She motioned me over to help the woman. I helped the woman make her way to the other side while Emily distracted her by chatting about how her daddy is used to heights because he works on the power lines.

We packed a lot into our few days there, even though Emily started to complain that her legs were hurting. Kari and I brushed off her complaints because she had been walking more than usual and we thought her legs were just tired. We thought she was just making excuses to sit down someplace where she could get ice cream. She was so energetic and excited by all the new things we were seeing. We didn't want her to start using this old excuse of her legs hurting as a way to get out of things the rest of the family wanted to do.

Later that month, Aunt Kathy, Kari's aunt on her mother's side, came to stay with Emily so Kari and I could have a date night. We were feeling good. Emily had been in remission for sixteen months, and in this mood of victory we asked each other questions we had not dared to ask when it seemed like Emily might not make it.

"Do you ever think, all of a sudden, oh my God, my daughter has cancer?" I asked Kari.

"Or just wake up in the middle of the night or stop in the middle of the aisle when you are grocery shopping and it hits you again?" Kari said.

I didn't know that she had the same physical reactions that I had, how when I thought those things my chest got tight and sometimes it felt like I couldn't breathe.

Kari compared that sensation to the moment when the doctor told her that Emily had cancer. Kari's first thoughts, after the shock subsided, were about all the people she knew, old and young, who had had leukemia and how they had suffered. Some of them had died. She feared how much Emily would suffer, and that she might not make it through. Kari also worried about me, she said, because stress causes flare-ups of my Crohn's disease, and if I got sick, too—well, she wasn't sure how she could handle that. As we sat at dinner, we appreciated that the most dire of those worries had not come to pass. On this date we had something to celebrate. We could talk about Emily's strong recovery and her joyful energy. She was still being treated for her cancer, of course. Our thoughts continued to be organized around that fact, but that night we took a few moments to acknowledge that everything was going as well as could be expected.

When we got home, Aunt Kathy greeted us at the door, but we could see right away that something was wrong. When Aunt Kathy told Emily it was time for bed, she'd asked why Lucy was lying over her legs. It was so unlike the energetic dog to be so still and quiet.

"Why doesn't she want to run and play, Emily?" Aunt Kathy asked.

"Because Lucy knows when I'm sick," Emily explained. "You know, Aunt Kathy, my blasts are growing again in my knees. In my blood and in my bones. The blasts are growing again."

Chapter 10

IT'S BACK

The blasts were back? How could this happen? Emily was full of energy and school was going well. Sometimes she came home tired, but after some downtime, she was ready to read or play. We'd just had a fantastic week in Vancouver, watching Emily run over the bridges and through the parks, chasing after the dogs in the hotel. How could the blasts be back? Dr. Powell recommended that we bring her in for a checkup and blood work just to be safe.

The next morning, as we were driving to the lab to get her blood drawn, I asked Emily how she knew the blasts were back.

"I felt the cancer pain in my knees again," Emily said. "I knew for sure it was back when Lucy didn't want to play and just laid beside me. Lucy let me know."

Lucy had a keen intuition. As a guy who likes to focus on the positive, I searched my memory for signs that Emily had beaten leukemia, that she had mustered her strength, and we had done everything the doctors told us to do. But as we drove to the appointment, I remembered those times in Vancouver when she'd complained she didn't want to walk because her knees hurt. I thought about how I'd had to persuade her to walk over that suspension bridge. The doctors had told me to stop carrying her and challenge her to get more activity to keep her strength up. *Tom,* I thought to myself, *remember, you must pay attention to the whispers.*

Normally it takes only a few hours to get the lab results back, but Dr. Powell didn't call that night, or leave a message, and it worried me and Kari. Maybe he had an emergency, Kari said. I agreed. He's the only pediatric oncologist at Mount Nittany Medical Center and when a family needs him, he is there for them.

What we didn't know was that he was checking and double-checking the results of the test. He'd examined a slide of Emily's blood but had seen just a few suspicious-looking cells. He knew the blood smear didn't tell the whole story, though, so he shared his results with a few of his colleagues. There had been several late-night chats between him and other doctors because he wanted to be sure before he alarmed us with bad news.

The next afternoon, I was at an executive board meeting for our union when I felt my phone vibrate and saw that it was Dr. Powell. I ducked out of the meeting to take his call.

"We do see a few blast cells," Dr. Powell said. "Over the past twenty-four hours I've had several other doctors review her blood smear under the microscope to make sure."

How will I tell Kari this? I thought.

"You need to go to Hershey right away," Dr. Powell said.

At home we explained to Emily that we had to go back to Hershey, and we couldn't promise she'd be back home for Halloween. She was not happy about this. Kari and she had just picked out her Halloween costume, a butterfly. They'd bought little butterfly clips to pin into her hair, which was growing back thick and wavy. I'd heard them planning how they were going to paint Emily's face so that she looked like a beautiful butterfly. Emily was sad all of that had to wait.

After Emily went to bed, Kari and I sat at the kitchen table. We were devastated to hear this news and terrified by what this could mean for Emily.

"I can't believe this is happening," Kari said.

"Hold on a second, Kari," I said. "We don't know for sure how serious this is yet. Dr. Powell said he only saw a few blasts in the blood smear."

"Ever since Emily was diagnosed, I thought she was going to be fine," Kari said. "I believed the doctors when they said she was going to be in the ninety percent of kids who beat leukemia. Why is this happening?"

"There were no warning signs," I said. "It wasn't like when she was first diagnosed when she had bruises and bleeding gums. We need to plan for the worst and pray for the best news."

Kari brought up the calendar on her phone and pointed to August 1, 2012, exactly twenty-six months from the day Emily was diagnosed.

"This was the day we could check leukemia off the list, and we could move on. We could put leukemia in the past. Now that she's relapsed, that day doesn't mean anything. We don't know how this will end, or when."

"Maybe the doctors at Hershey will contradict Dr. Powell," I said.

"The doctors kept telling us that we were doing everything right," Kari said. "We never missed an appointment or chemotherapy."

"This isn't our fault," I said, pulling Kari in for a hug.

"That makes it even scarier," Kari said. "It shows us how aggressive this cancer is."

———— ··◉·· ————

The next day at Hershey, Dr. Ungar ordered more blood work and tested the strength in Emily's legs to make sure there wasn't any sign of infection developing again. He pressed his palms on the soles of her feet and told her to resist his push, which she did with a lot of force. He grinned at her strength, and at us.

"I don't know, Tom, Kari," he said. "This feels like a false alarm. She's strong, no bruising, no sign of infection. I'm not seeing blast cells in the blood work we just did here. We'll look at her bone marrow just to be safe."

Twenty minutes after the bone marrow aspiration, he came back.

"Her bone marrow," he said. "It's full of cancer."

———————

Emily had one of the worst types of relapse because she was still in treatment and receiving chemotherapy. This meant that the cancer had become resistant to standard therapies. The only treatment available, the one that had had the most success over time, was a bone marrow transplant. To qualify for one, Emily would have to get into remission again, which meant that she would need to go through several months of more intense chemotherapy. The doctors told us it would be more difficult to get her into remission this time, and the chemotherapy would make her sicker than before. When we asked about her chance of being cured with a bone marrow transplant, they told us that only 30 percent of children who have a transplant are alive five years later. I was having a hard time containing the sorrow that was rising in me, but I kept it down by focusing on holding Kari's hand and praying.

The protocol for bone marrow transplant sounded grueling as the doctors described the "roadmap" for the next four months. They talked about the phases of Emily's treatment, the "blocks" of chemo she would get, and how the way her body responded to each phase would determine what happened next. Over the next three months, she'd get three blocks of successively stronger chemo, then she'd have a month to recover before she got the transplant.

Emily would receive healthy blood cells from an anonymous donor. Before receiving the cells, she would need an additional ten days of high-dose chemotherapy and full-body radiation. This process is called conditioning and the purpose is to wipe out her bone marrow to make room for these healthy donor cells to grow. After Emily received the cells, Kari and I would be with Emily in her hospital room for four to six weeks waiting for the cells to settle into her bone marrow and start growing. Since her immune system would be wiped out, she would not be allowed to leave her room and visitors would be restricted because her body would not be able to fight off viruses or infections. If she survived that, our family would live for a month or two in an apartment in Hershey because we couldn't be more than ten minutes from the hospital in case she developed complications. If all of this stayed on track, with no setbacks, we might be able to go back home sometime in May. Maybe that should be the new date in Kari's calendar: that we could be home in time for Emily's seventh birthday on May 2.

Kari and I tried to wrap our minds around how we would be with Emily during this long period where she would need our constant attention. On CaringBridge, Kari followed many families whose child had a bone marrow transplant. She knew of a few children who, despite horrendous odds and many setbacks, made it through and were cancer free after the transplant. There were many more devastating endings, though. We were praying that Emily would be part of that 30 percent but, from what Kari knew of the other families' stories, the odds didn't look good. The suffering we knew she would have to endure over the next few months was unbearable to think about.

Already the mood in the room was somber. Everything hung on finding the right donor for Emily. They started a search for a donor through an international bone marrow registry. We had nothing to do but wait to see if someone who matched with Emily was ready to donate. Kari posted on the blog that we needed people to pray for Emily, writing she just didn't know how to believe anymore that Emily was going to be okay. I felt terrible about that. Hope was my job, and I was failing at it if Kari was discouraged.

Kari's way of dealing with the situation was to learn as much as she could about relapsed leukemia. I saw her grab the laptop to research bone marrow transplants. When Emily first got sick, Kari always took careful notes when we spoke to the doctors and searched for information to see if she could advance her knowledge beyond what they told her, but she never doubted their judgment. With a 90 percent cure rate, there wasn't much reason to question the doctors. With the relapse, Kari was determined to find the best route to a cure for Emily.

In the hospital, Emily was withdrawn much of the time, except when we tried to get her to FaceTime with Lucy, which was hilarious. Lucy didn't quite understand what was going on. She started licking the phone, which made Emily giggle. It worried me that this time Emily wasn't interested in her illness, not feisty or sassy. Like us, she'd thought she was close to being done with treatment. It was as if she didn't understand why we were back at Hershey when we had kept telling her she was beating cancer. I didn't know how to tell her what was ahead of her with the bone marrow transplant, even though she'd been there when we were talking to the doctors about it. She didn't meet the doctors' eyes when they described the treatment and she didn't ask any questions.

Nurse Karli to the rescue!

Nurse Karli came into Emily's room with a pad of paper and some markers and pulled a chair up next to Emily's bed. She handed some of the markers to Emily and asked her to help her draw a colorful garden. When they'd filled the page with bright flowers, Nurse Karli began the story.

"In a healthy garden there were lots of flowers and not very many weeds. In the bone marrow garden, the good cells that make the blood are the flowers and the bad cells are the weeds."

Nurse Karli drew some frowning plants and some angry ones, the evil weeds.

"Sometimes when there are too many weeds in the garden, we have to spray it with chemo to kill off the weeds that are trying to take over the garden," she said. Nurse Karli drew a spray bottle blasting out a cone of lines over the weedy garden.

"When the weed spray is not enough, when there are still too many weeds, we have to pull up the whole garden and get new soil and replant it with new seeds. That's what the bone marrow transplant is. The doctors are replanting the garden with new soil to grow big, bright flowers again."

"Will it make me as sick as before?" Emily asked.

"When the garden is starting to grow again, germs can make you sick," Nurse Karli said. "The good news is that while the garden is starting to grow again, Mom and Dad will stay with you and play games and watch television to keep you safe and happy. You get anything you need while the garden gets thick with flowers. I will be there, too, if you have any questions, or if your tummy starts to hurt. I've got something to help with that."

This was such a hard time for us, and it really helped to feel the support of so many competent and compassionate people like Nurse Karli, who described the care and support Emily would receive so that the whole thing wouldn't seem so scary. We were feeling that support, too—in the hospital, and coming from the thousands of people reading Kari's blog.

What was different during this hospital stay was that our community from the blog had grown so much larger. We had thousands of people following Kari's writing every day, and, when Emily relapsed, there were many more. Kari posted our room number on the blog and we started receiving dozens of cards daily from her followers, mostly for Halloween, and they sent candy and decorations, too. One of the nurses paused for a few minutes to take a look at the dozens of cards and letters we had pinned to the walls, over the bed, all around, a riot of autumn colors. Intermixed with all those good wishes for Emily's recovery were pictures of Lucy scampering around at home. The people who followed Emily's story were in love with the photos of Lucy, too. One of them paid for an artist in California to make an exact stuffed-animal replica of Lucy so Emily could snuggle with her dog even though they were separated. Emily loved the way Kari had decorated the walls, but we couldn't help comparing this Halloween to the last one.

Instead of being able to style her hair with those butterfly clips, we shaved Emily's head again because the nurses said she would lose her hair quickly this time. Kari had to take the elastic out of Emily's butterfly costume because it was too tight on her chest port, so it sagged. Kari hadn't brought the fancy makeup. Emily had to wear a green mask to protect her from germs in the hospital air, so no one could really see her face anyway. Nurse Karli tried to boost Emily's spirits by giving her a bottle of glitter to sprinkle on her forehead and her hands. Emily thanked her but she didn't smile or laugh as she handed it back to Kari.

We pushed Emily in a wagon down the hall, her IV pole trailing behind her, extending a candy bag to everyone who walked by and going in and out of the department offices where the staff had bags of miniature

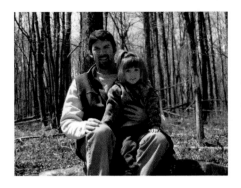

Tom and Emily at camp before diagnosis (age three).

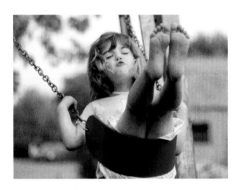

Emily swinging on the swing set Tom built (age four).

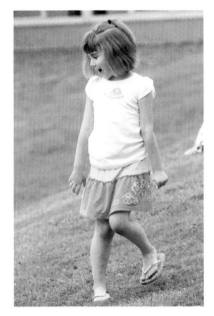

Emily two weeks before diagnosis (age five). We went back through photos after she was diagnosed and noticed that in this photo she has bruises on her legs, so she would have had leukemia at this time but we didn't know yet.

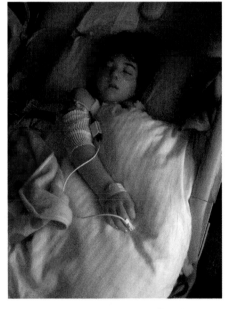

At Hershey Medical Center a few days after diagnosis.

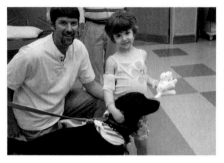

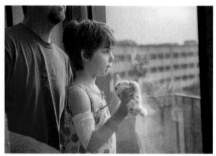

At Hershey Medical Center with Jasper the therapy dog after her haircut. She has the PICC line in her arm.

At Hershey Medical Center. She has the PICC line in her arm. Tom is in the background.

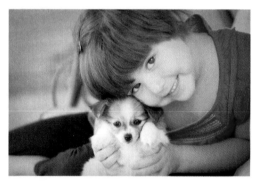

Emily and Lucy.

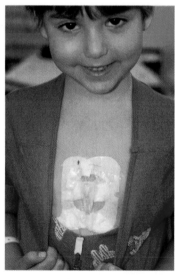

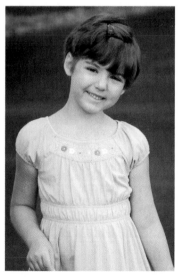

Emily with her Mediport.

Emily's first day of kindergarten.

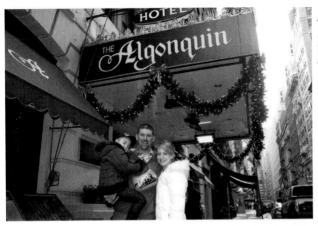
Tom, Kari, and Emily in NYC at the Algonquin Hotel.

Emily shaving Tom's head in the hospital

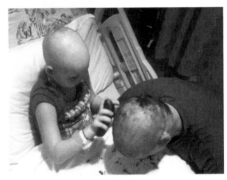

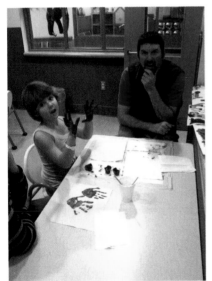

Waiting in the oncology outpatient clinic at Hershey Medical Center after Emily relapsed. Child life specialists kept the kids busy during the long days of appointments and treatments.

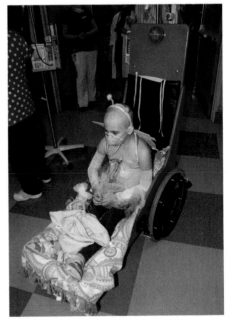

Emily in her butterfly costume trick-or-treating in the hospital.

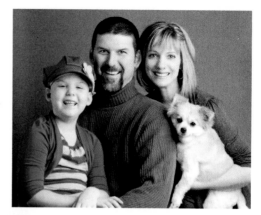

Tom, Kari, Emily, and Lucy.

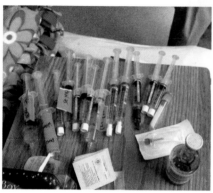

The typical number of medications that Emily would get through her IV at one particular time of the day. (This would be repeated several times a day.)

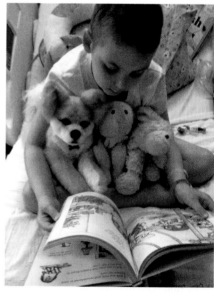

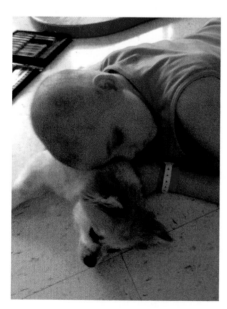

Lucy's visit to Hershey Medical Center.

Emily passing the time, reading her book to her stuffed animals (including the stuffed Lucy dog)—long days at CHOP waiting for the CAR T cells to be ready. She was very sick from chemo here.

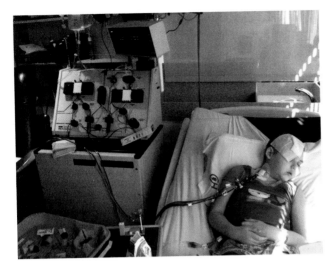

Emily connected to the apheresis machine to remove the T cells from her blood.

CAR–T cell infusion day! Dr. Grupp giving Emily the CAR T cells.

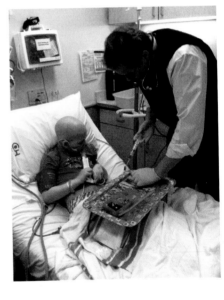

Tom and Kari holding Emily's hand while Emily fought for her life in the PICU.

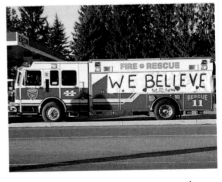

Community support at a prayer vigil.

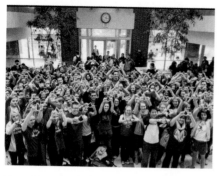

Penn State students who sang an early "Happy Birthday" to Emily in the HUB.

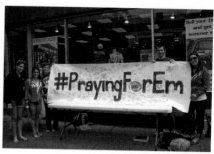

The banner Becky and Ariana made and had people sign outside the student bookstore.

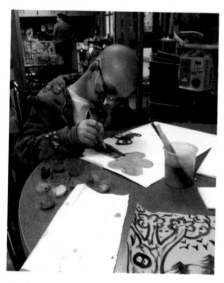

Emily in the art room at CHOP, painting and recovering after being in the PICU.

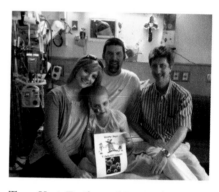

Tom, Kari, Emily, and Dr. Bruce Levine the day before we left CHOP to come home.

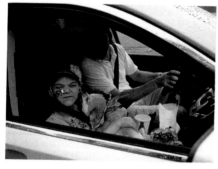

Homecoming—Lucy licking Emily's face and greeting her.

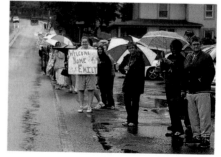

Homecoming—people standing outside in the rain, waiting to see us drive through town and bring Emily home.

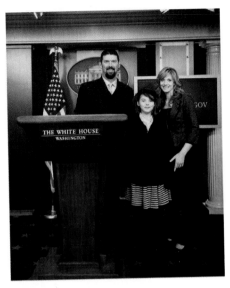

At the White House the day we met
Barack Obama.

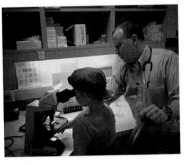

Dr. Powell showing Emily what
leukemia cells look like under a
microscope.

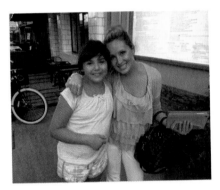

Emily with Nurse Karli.

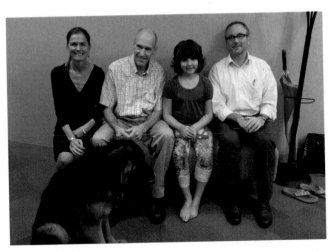

Emily with Dr. June (to her right), Dr. Kalos (to her left), and
Dr. June's wife, Lisa (and their dog Lacey!), when we stopped
to visit Dr. June at his office at Penn Medicine.

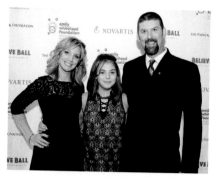

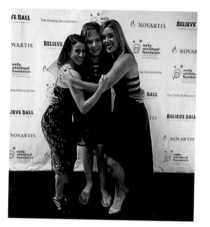

Tom, Kari, and Emily at the Emily Whitehead Foundation Believe Ball—our first gala that raised over $450,000 for pediatric cancer research.

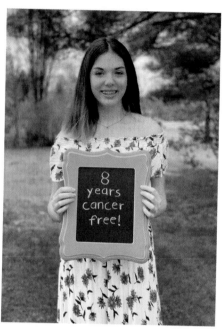

Emily with Becky and Ariana at the Emily Whitehead Foundation Believe Ball.

Eight years cancer-free.

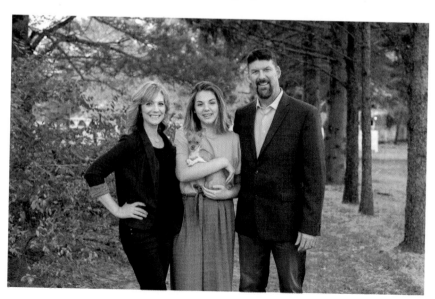

Most recent family photo: Tom, Kari, Emily, and Luna.

candy bars for the kids. She was getting a lot of candy, but it felt like a chore. Kari's mood matched Emily's. Last year Kari wrote on the blog about how great the staff was to make such an effort for these kids. This year, because Emily's odds had changed so dramatically, Kari felt as though people in the hallway were staring at us. Many passersby had kindly eyes, but others stared with pity. Emily's mood improved when we got back to the room and she poured her mountain of candy on the bed to sort through all she'd acquired. Also, when we got back, she received a dose of steroids. That plus the candy had her talking a mile a minute.

> While I've been writing this Emily has been talking to me nonstop and asking all kinds of random questions, such as "How old is SpongeBob?" and "How exactly does my letter to Santa get to his house? Is there really a post office at the North Pole?" We never know what her mood will be like when she is on steroids. Earlier she would not say a word to anyone and now she's chatting away with everyone who walks into the room. Except for the doctors—she completely ignores them. She won't even look at them when they come in the room. They ask her a question and she just pretends they aren't there. Occasionally she will say "Meep!" which is her code word for "Leave me alone. It doesn't matter how long you stand here and try talking to me. I will just totally pretend you are not there."
>
> —Kari's journal
> October 31, 2011

Kari was determined that we needed to get a second opinion. Although we were always very happy with the care Emily received at Hershey, we felt we should also consult with a larger hospital. As I knew from my health issues, a second opinion is always a good idea. You never know what additional information you might learn. Kari mentioned a few hospitals that were within driving distance—Pittsburgh Children's, Johns Hopkins, and Children's Hospital of Philadelphia.

Kari filled out an online form requesting a second opinion on the website for Children's Hospital of Philadelphia (CHOP), which had a reputation as a great research hospital. The next morning, I got a call from Dr. Susan Rheingold, one of the top doctors in the country who treats relapsed childhood leukemia. I was so impressed that she called me right away.

She asked us to send Emily's medical records, so we got them printed out. That was quite a stack! We went to UPS to send off this huge package. Dr. Rheingold said she would review the records, and she advised us to make an appointment to see her at CHOP as soon as possible.

Philadelphia is a long four hours from Philipsburg. I was thinking as we drove there a few days later how it was already tough on our families to drive the two hours to Hershey. We'd see a lot less of them if we set up Emily's care in Philadelphia. Also, Emily was comfortable at Hershey, and so were we. We knew the staff well. We trusted and respected the doctors, and we loved the nurses and our THON family. It was important that Emily feel solid and grounded no matter what the disease threw her way.

CHOP is at the southeastern edge of Philadelphia, right against the Schuylkill River, surrounded by Penn Medicine, the University of Pennsylvania, and other medical facilities and research labs. We made our way through dozens of taxis and cars and ambulances crowded onto a street where families pushed their loved ones of all ages in wheelchairs through the sliding glass doors in search of healing. I'd never felt that kind of energy on a street before, such a concentrated yearning. Yet when we walked into CHOP, I felt hope. We entered an atrium seven stories tall, filled with light. To our left was a playful perpetual-motion sculpture, constantly chiming as colorful balls traveled down chutes and ratcheted up on conveyor belts, hitting the bells along the way. And there was a recording studio where a young patient was singing solo to her favorite song backed by a karaoke machine.

We met with Dr. Rheingold, a soft-spoken woman with warm, deep-brown eyes who reassures you just by being in the room. She seemed to have answers to all our questions and already had several plans in place for treating Emily. After reviewing Emily's records, she said they saw no indicators as to why she'd relapsed; she should have been in the 90 percent who do not. She agreed with Hershey that a bone marrow transplant was the next best treatment for Emily, and emphasized that CHOP's approach would be similar, and she hoped it worked. If it did not, the advantage at CHOP was what came after that. As a leading research hospital, CHOP is often able to offer cutting-edge treatments to children. The doctors conduct clinical research trials on the latest approaches to treating disease, allowing them to bring the newest therapies to the children treated at CHOP.

Kari wanted to know more about these new treatments and if Emily would be eligible for any clinical trials. Dr. Rheingold said it was an individual decision based on the patient. The delicate balance for the doctors was to make sure to preserve as many treatment options for the patient as they could. The qualifications for including a child in a clinical trial are precise. Maybe one clinical trial specified it would only include patients who had not had a bone marrow transplant, or it excluded those who had taken a particular kind of chemo. The very things we might try to save Emily's life could prevent her from being in a clinical trial.

While Kari and Dr. Rheingold discussed more of the scientific specifics, I took Emily on a walk around the children's cancer floor, guided by another doctor, Dr. Nancy Bunin. The cancer floor had much bigger rooms than we had at Hershey, and I liked that. As we walked out of one of the patient rooms and turned back to join Kari, I stopped in my tracks when I saw the hallway leading to the bone marrow transplant unit.

To my eyes, the hallway was glowing. I envisioned myself there with Emily. She was pale and weak, but she had beaten cancer. She was taking small steps with a walker, and she seemed very tired. I had my arm around her, and she was leaning on me. It seemed as if I were teaching her how to walk again in that hallway.

The vision struck me like one of my whispers, but I didn't understand it. This seemed like a vision from the future, as my whispers often do. Or maybe it was a one-off, not a whisper but a hallucination, because I desperately needed a sign of something to hope for. I decided not to tell Kari about the vision in the hallway because I couldn't trust what it was just yet.

We decided that if both hospitals were going to treat Emily's cancer the same way, it was better for her, better for all of us, to be closer to our family. We thanked Dr. Rheingold and left.

We settled back in at Hershey, where we knew the staff and had our family and friends close by, praying for that bone marrow donor to come through soon.

———··●··———

It was interesting to me how close Kari and I had become with Becky and Ariana in the last year. They had become part of our emotional support group, calling us to find out how Emily was doing, and serving as a shoulder to cry on when we didn't feel we could burden our parents with more to worry about. With Becky and Ariana, we could explore our fears and our hopes without them advocating for one solution or another, although both were very much on board with the idea of getting a second opinion at CHOP.

My family has very strong opinions about everything and, while they meant the best for us, sometimes when they were expressing a strong sentiment about what we should do, the conversation would start to sound like an argument. What Kari and I needed was to hear our own hearts speaking out loud about what might be the next best step for Emily. With Ariana and Becky, because they were young and didn't feel they could advise us, we had people who would let us just vent or allow us to express our confusion without pressuring us to make decisions before we were ready. At this point we were so frightened and confused that we honestly didn't know what to do.

Our worry now was how to decide between Hershey and CHOP—comfort versus the chance for something new. Was it better for Emily to be close to home and be able to see people who loved her nearly every day? Did that support mean more than access to cutting-edge treatments?

The son of one of the families we had met at Hershey had recently passed away from leukemia. They had transferred to CHOP when things started to go downhill for the boy. They told us later that the one regret they had was that they had not transferred to CHOP sooner because they felt if they had, he might still be alive. There is no way of knowing that, of course, and we loved the doctors and the care that we got at Hershey. Yet that opinion hung in my mind while we considered whether we needed a third or even a fourth opinion.

In keeping Emily comfortable and surrounded by family, was she missing out on some new medical advance that could save her life? Kari was the most torn up about this. I kept thinking CHOP was someplace up ahead in Emily's future, though that vision I'd had with Emily and me in the bone marrow transplant hallway had not come back. *Focus on the here and now until the whispers get louder and I understand them more,* I thought.

Hershey discharged Emily and we went back home at the end of her first block of chemo. I went back to work, and Kari stayed home with Emily. The only thing Kari wanted to do was to sit on the couch with Emily and watch cartoons, to keep the house tidy, and cook our own food. Kari, eagle-eyed for germs, found super-strong antiseptic wipes that were so powerful they had a toxic warning symbol on the container. Kari had to wear gloves when she used them to wipe down the grocery store cart. That's how vigilant we thought we had to be as we waited for the latest blood work results that would show how Emily had responded to that first block of chemo.

We did not receive the news we wanted. We just heard from Hershey. We knew something was wrong since it has taken them 24 hours to get back to us. Usually they can tell within an hour of the bone marrow aspiration if there is remission. There are still a lot of immature cells in Emily's marrow. They can't tell with the microscope if they are actual blast cells. They are sending it away for more testing. It's possible they are just immature good cells, but it sounds like they feel she still has 4–5% blast cells. With that many blast cells the bone marrow transplant is unlikely to work.

—Kari's Journal
November 9, 2011

After the news that the first block of chemotherapy was not as effective as we had needed it to be for her to qualify for a bone marrow transplant,

Emily seemed exhausted. Some days she only wanted to lie on the sofa watching TV with Lucy. We could see that cancer was sucking the life out of her and out of us. The psychologist at Hershey told us that kids never give up. But Kari knew from reading stories of other cancer families that children know when their time has come. They start talking about dying. We feared Emily might give up, and we didn't know what we would do then. Right around that time, Emily asked, "What will I do if my cancer keeps coming back?"

"We will keep fighting it," Kari said.

Just when we thought there was no good news to be had, we found out on November 11 that Emily actually *was* in remission! The cells they saw were just immature good cells and not cancer cells, as they had originally thought. Emily had fewer than 1 percent cancer cells in her blood, which made her eligible for a bone marrow transplant if the cancer cells stayed at that percentage. We were so happy with this news, which we got the day before Emily was scheduled to begin the second block of chemo, a tough one that would require her to be admitted to the hospital for more than a week. It looked like we were going to spend Thanksgiving in the hospital, so before we left for Hershey, I watched Kari take down all the Halloween decorations and put up the Christmas stuff, skipping over Thanksgiving.

"We're focusing on Christmas," Kari said. "We'll be home for Christmas."

Chapter 11

---·•◦•·---

HOW CAN WE SAVE EMILY?

Hershey keeps all the T cells...CHOP keeps a few T cells. What does this mean for Emily and the outcome of the transplant? No one can tell us. All we know is that the bone marrow from the donor is processed differently and there isn't any answer as to which way is better. We are trying to understand and make a decision about something that takes medical school plus an additional 7+ years of being a doctor to fully understand. It's stressful and frustrating and we still don't know the answer. Each hospital tells us that doing it their way is better for Emily.

—Kari's Journal
November 16, 2011

Kari's instincts were right about Thanksgiving. We were out of the hospital for a few days after that first dose of Block 2 chemo, but then Emily got chills and spiked a fever during a clinic visit, so they admitted her, thinking she might have an infection. They didn't want to take any chances. We got a three-hour pass to leave the hospital to have Thanksgiving dinner with Aunt Laurie and the cousins, and we were glad for the break, but it was clear Emily wouldn't be discharged anytime soon. Her ANC (absolute neutrophil count), which measures the number of infection-fighting white blood cells she has, was 50, essentially zero; a healthy count ranges from 1,500 to 8,000. The harsh chemo also made her nauseous and gave her mouth sores, making it difficult for her to eat. Her oxygen levels kept dipping below 90 percent when she slept, so they kept her on oxygen at night.

Kari and I were worried, but Emily was sassy and feisty around that time. If anyone irritated her, she would write their name on a dry-erase board, give them detention, and order them out of the room. When Pappy Rob came to visit, he said or did something that rubbed her the wrong way. He was not allowed to talk to her at all, only permitted to follow her orders. "Get me a drink!" she instructed him. "Take me to the playroom!"

Of course we were talking a lot about the bone marrow transplant, but Emily never said much about it. She must have heard us discuss the fact that if she received marrow from a male donor, a blood test would show that she was a male. One day, out of the blue, she had a question.

"So, if I get cells from a boy does that mean I am going to turn into a boy?" she asked.

"No!" I said, chuckling.

"But then I could pee standing up!" she said. She has an amazing ability to turn things around.

We were disappointed when her ANC was still only 50 after Thanksgiving, but a few days later her ANC was 6,600, high enough that they let her go home. We wanted to cram in as many Christmas activities as we could because we never knew if Emily would end up spending the holiday in the hospital. We went to the Philipsburg Christmas parade, and the THON students paid us a visit. Becky brought four other THON friends with her, and they played Emily's favorite game: animals. She assigned each one of them an animal. The students then had to act like that animal, making animal noises, crawling all over the house, jumping from the ottoman to the couch, begging for food. It was very funny to see college kids pretending to be cats and dogs, wagging their tails and licking their paws. Then suddenly Emily got pain in her right side, started vomiting, and we had to go to the ER at around 11:00 p.m. on a Saturday night.

From October through January, we lived in the hospital most of the time. We were able to come home only for a few days before Emily spiked a fever, or needed a blood or platelet transfusion, or she had to be readmitted for chemotherapy. We were anxious as we watched her lab values fluctuate.

For us, 2012 will start off either good or bad, depending on how you look at it. On one hand Emily will get a bone marrow transplant that we hope will save her life. But on the other hand...well, Emily is getting a bone marrow transplant. We hope this turns into a wonderful year for us. 2010 brought cancer. 2011 brought more cancer. How about 2012 brings a cure?

—Kari's journal
December 31, 2011

The good news was that there were many potential bone marrow donors for Emily. There were several who were a ten-out-of-ten match for specific proteins on her cells, meaning that the donor's cells should settle in Emily's bone marrow with fewer complications. We were overjoyed to learn this, and grateful to the donor they chose, whom we hoped to meet one day. The donor remains anonymous until a year after the transplant, and they put you in touch only if both the patient and the donor agree.

Once we had a match, the focus was keeping Emily in remission until the transplant, which was scheduled for early February. That first week in February, if all went according to plan, the donor would come in to a hospital to have stem cells harvested in a procedure similar to donating blood. The technicians at that hospital would package up those cells and ship them to Hershey, where Emily would receive them through an infusion. The cells would then migrate to her bone marrow, where they would settle in to begin growing healthy blood cells.

That date for the bone marrow transplant kept moving because the donor needed to delay. The transplant was initially scheduled for February 7, but on January 6 the doctors told us there would be a two-week delay, which meant it wouldn't happen until February 21. We never knew the reason for these delays, and I was having a hard time containing my frustration because this was delaying Emily's recovery. Did this person sign up to donate bone marrow to save a stranger's life because it sounded like a noble thing to do and then get cold feet when the day came to make the donation? I did not know. I wanted to continue to be grateful to this person because he or she might be the person who saved Emily's life. Yet they must not have understood how fragile this moment was, how we needed to be able to act quickly. And then the donor delayed again, until February 28.

Emily seemed oblivious to these delays, so I guess Kari and I were hiding our anxiety well enough. The fact that she was on a large dose of steroids made her fierce at air hockey; she wanted to go to the playroom at least once a day, and she was beating me! I teased her that it wasn't fair because she was on performance-enhancing drugs. Inside I was dying from the tension and from being cooped up in the hospital with no way to improve Emily's chances of survival.

We were on our way home from Hershey after the most recent hospital stay, driving in two cars, with me in the lead. Emily was not feeling well and we wanted to get home quickly, so I told Kari I'd go faster than her. If there were police along the way who caught us speeding, they'd snag me, and she and Emily could keep going. We were coming into State College with only about twenty-five miles until we were home. I didn't see the officer sitting in the median. Kari was the one who got pulled over. He could have stopped me, but he went for the cute blond instead.

I pulled off ahead of Kari, then the officer was right behind her.

I opened my driver's-side window and shouted, "Officer, can I speak to you? I'm the husband. We have a sick child. Can you talk to me first?"

He heard me and ignored what I said. He started asking Kari for her identification.

"He'll see Emily," I tried to reassure myself. "He'll see she's bald and those dark circles under her eyes and he'll let Kari go."

I felt I had to check on Emily, but my state trooper friends have told me never to approach a policeman or patrol car during a traffic stop. I shouted again as he walked smugly back to the patrol car to check Kari's license and registration, again ignoring me.

I couldn't take it anymore. I know a lot of the state troopers at this local barracks, and I could let him know that I was not a threat. I opened my car door and slowly walked to the passenger side of Kari's vehicle. I opened the back door to make sure Emily wasn't frightened. I saw that Emily was sleeping, and again, I tried to get the officer's attention. He clearly heard me but ignored me. I wanted to let him know that Emily was sick and we needed to get her home. I took two steps in his direction.

He immediately got out of his car and started screaming at me.

"You go back to your car right now!" he yelled.

He put his hand on his weapon as if he was going to draw on me.

I returned to my vehicle.

I passed the time he took reviewing Kari's paperwork by calling my state trooper friend Gary, who calmed me down. When the officer returned from handing Kari a warning, he finally walked to my passenger-side window to acknowledge me.

"Is that your family?" he asked.

"That is. That's my daughter sick with cancer."

"You can't come at my car," he said. "That's a threat to me."

"Can't you see she's extremely sick? You could have given me the ticket. You should have let them go!"

"I could tell you have a sick child. I only gave them a warning," he said.

"I hope that you never have to experience having a sick child," I said, and then pulled out.

When we arrived home, Emily was giggling.

"Daddy, I pretended I was asleep while Mommy was being arrested, but I was sleep-listening," she said.

Leave it to Emily to get us to smile that day.

Maybe I would have handled that situation better if I had not been feeling the stress of it all in every cell of my body. The next time Emily was admitted at Hershey, I was, too. The tension caused my Crohn's disease to flare up and I was in agony. I had arranged to get my infusion of Remicade at Hershey, a procedure that takes a few hours. The Remicade is expensive and they don't mix it up until you arrive at the infusion suite. Before they start the infusion, they check your vital signs, your heart rate, blood pressure, and temperature. While I was getting my infusion, I got a fever and they thought I might be getting an infection, so they admitted me to the hospital. This upset me even more; the anxiety that comes from futility. I would be in this hospital room far away from Kari and Emily. If something went wrong suddenly, I couldn't be there for them.

The staff at Hershey was so kind to us. Emily's room faced a courtyard and they put me in a room a few floors down from her, a room visible from her window. She used the binoculars to look at me, and we spoke on the phone even if it was just for us to shout "Meep!" I was soothed by being able to see her whenever I wanted. The hospital really helped us make the best of it.

> Nothing feels right, we are second-guessing all of our decisions, and we are pretty much starting to totally freak out about every-thing right now....Please pray for no fever and no infections for Emily and that her counts come up and we can go home soon!
>
> —Kari's journal
> January 11, 2012

Being in limbo, with the lab numbers fluctuating and the uncertainty about when the transplant would happen, had us pacing the hallways. Anytime we wanted to take a phone call, we'd have to leave the room because we didn't want Emily to hear us say what we were thinking. Mostly Emily was fine, but it was agony for me and Kari. Should we take her to CHOP? No, no. They would be doing exactly what Hershey was doing, so why change? But was there something else there that could save Emily? I was sleeping on the bench in Emily's room when another vision of the bone marrow transplant hallway jolted me awake. Me and Emily, my arm around her, strong and determined, taking one slow step after another. Was this a sign? Should we defy the doctors, and all the logic, and just drive to CHOP?

Since we were just waiting, there was no reason to make a move. We were home for quite a while at the end of January and able to have visitors, which took our minds off some of our worries. Kari took Emily for routine blood work at a local lab on February 2 and drove over to get the results as soon as they were available. She immediately called me.

"I think it's back. Her white blood cell count is nineteen thousand," Kari said, her voice shaking. The normal range is between 4,500 and 10,500.

We called Dr. Powell, who said that when he reviewed the blood work, he hadn't seen any blast cells. He only saw a lot of immature white cells, which could mean the bone marrow was making new blood cells. He recommended we get blood work again in two days. On February 4, Dr. Powell called while we were at Pappy Rob's for dinner to tell us we needed to take Emily to Hershey in the morning. Her white blood cell count had shot up to 46,000 with 33 percent blasts. My chest tightened in fear as Dr. Powell told me this information. We knew what it meant. Emily had relapsed again.

———————•••••——————

That first night back at Hershey, I had an upset stomach, and I thought, *There is no way I can get sick right now. I can't let the Crohn's flare up again. It would take me out of the fight, and I need to be there for Emily.* I had to get out of Emily's room, though. It felt like I was spreading my pain to Emily and Kari, and they were starting to worry about me.

I went to spend the night at the Ronald McDonald House, which is a fantastic resource for parents of sick children, offering free or low-cost lodging for parents who are staying near the hospital while their children get treated. In my room there, I was touching my Saint Christopher medal from my grandmother. When she gave it to me, she'd said that she was praying for me and that she knew this medal would guide me out of my disease, and it had been my talisman the whole time Emily was sick. When I touched it, I felt closer to my grandmother's spirit of love and faith, and I could hear my whispers more clearly.

I knelt beside the bed to pray, thinking how this bone marrow transplant had to happen. I asked the good Lord to influence the donor to stop with the delays, to find it in his or her heart to put our Emily first. I wanted God to guide the actions of this stranger to save Emily, to save our family. And that night, the vision in the bone marrow transplant hallway happened again—the same thing—and I woke up and thought, *Well, people say they get a sign. Here's my sign. She's going to get better at CHOP. We're going to be teaching her to walk again. We're going to be in the bone marrow transplant hallway.*

Early the next morning, before I got to Hershey, Dr. Lucas and Dr. Freiberg were in a rush to present a new treatment plan to Kari. With this second relapse, there was no standard treatment protocol to follow. They had to use their best judgment to see if any combination of chemotherapies would get Emily back into remission so she could proceed to transplant.

"We need to get something started for Emily right away," Dr. Lucas said. "Her white blood cell count is increasing rapidly. Her organs may start to fail."

"We agreed that we're going to give her a round of chemotherapy called ICE. It's three different drugs: ifosfamide, carboplatin, and etoposide," Dr. Lucas said. "It's really intense chemo. She hasn't had anything like it. There is a risk of developing neurotoxicity and kidney failure. I just want you to be prepared."

Kari reached me in the dining room at the Ronald McDonald House.

"Tom, you have to get over here right now. The doctors want give her a combination of drugs, and it doesn't feel right to me."

I got a sick feeling in the pit of my stomach when I arrived at the hospital room and overheard the two doctors arguing over the treatment. If they couldn't agree, why would we consider it?

"Tom and I need to talk about this alone," Kari said.

"Okay," said Dr. Lucas. "I'll have the pharmacy begin preparing the chemo."

"Not yet," I said. "Kari and I want to talk about this."

The doctors left the room and Kari turned to me. She'd already made up her mind.

"I am really uncomfortable with this plan. It just doesn't feel right," she said. "I think we need to go back to CHOP."

"I agree," I said.

As we were starting the process of getting Emily discharged, Dr. Freiberg came into the room to try to persuade us not to go.

"She's not stable enough to transfer," Dr. Freiberg said.

"Our instincts tell us we have to get another opinion," I said.

"There are no more second opinions," Dr. Freiberg said. "She needs to start chemo now, or you're putting her life at risk."

"If you feel she's not stable, get a helicopter," I said. "I don't care if we have to pay for it. We're taking her to CHOP for another opinion."

"I can tell you what's going to happen," Dr. Freiberg said. "You're going to take her to CHOP and they will treat her in an experimental trial."

I didn't want to hear this.

"When you get there, a young doctor is going to offer you a Phase 1 clinical trial that's not going to do anything to help Emily. They're going to use her body to figure out the right dose of a new medicine and she will suffer. It won't do anything to help her."

"We've already made up our minds," I said.

"Then you are doing this against doctors' orders," Dr. Freiberg said.

"I respect you, Dr. Freiberg," I said. "I'm not telling you what we're doing tomorrow. All I can tell you is we're going to CHOP right now."

It was like we had to fight our way out of the hospital and onto the turnpike to Philadelphia. Everywhere we looked we saw danger and doubt, and we couldn't be sure we were doing the right thing. By the time we were halfway to Philadelphia, Emily was asleep, and Kari finally let herself cry.

"What do I know? I'm just a mom," Kari said. "The doctors know what they are doing. They scared me so much when they started arguing in front of me. Maybe I'm just having a mom reaction. Maybe she does need the ICE chemo. Maybe we need to do what they say."

I didn't want to chime in about the whispers. I was watching her make up her mind, and what I needed to do was listen to her, not them.

"We need to educate ourselves so we can make the best decision for Emily," she concluded, becoming more confident in our decision as we got closer to CHOP.

"That's what we're doing," I agreed.

We met heavy traffic the entire way. When it slowed to a stop, I was berating myself, taking personal responsibility for the traffic. Emily had to go to the bathroom, so I pulled over to a big chain restaurant, a sit-down-dinner kind of place. I gathered Emily up, her body limp from the morphine. The hostess blanched when she saw us. Seeing Emily through a stranger's eyes jolted me. Day by day it could seem reasonable enough. We were managing. We were doing what we were told and focused on the best outcome. Could I no longer see how sick Emily was because I was so focused on her survival?

Back in the car, back on the turnpike, I got chest pains looking at her sleeping in the backseat. I thought, *Am I making the wrong decision for my child? Is she going to die because we're changing hospitals?*

We got admitted to CHOP, and we were just getting settled in Emily's new room when a young doctor came in to offer us a Phase 1 clinical trial, just like Dr. Freiberg predicted.

"This is what we have open today," he said. "It's a chemotherapy she's never had called temsirolimus."

It was unfamiliar to Kari. She told the doctor we needed time to think. As soon as the doctor left, she opened her laptop to begin researching the drug. I took this chance to take another look at the bone marrow transplant hallway.

I had such a firm image of it from the distortions of my visions and dreams. In my visions I always saw it first as if I were looking into the hallway at the two figures moving there, me and Emily. And from this vantage point it was a place that glowed. After that, the view was a close-up of Emily, of me holding her with one arm around her torso, her on her walker with the tennis balls to smooth the way and the noisemakers on her heels that let out a big *eep* every time her heel hit the floor. Emily was pale, much paler than she had been when she was stomping around last year at home on her walker, but she was all Emily. All gumption and spirit and with that incredible will to live. And in the vision, I was not the broken and terrified father lurching through the world trying to decide the right thing to do. I was full of gratitude in a place without time. My daughter was weak, but healing, and it would take however long it took to get her healthy again. She knew I'd always be at her side.

With this vision in my mind, I turned the corner to the hallway, and it didn't match my vision at all. Maybe one of the lights was out, but it seemed dim and depressing. The parents in the hallway looked exhausted. Try as I might to project me and Emily into that space, I couldn't do it. I couldn't see us there. I was even more confused than before. This vision I had been tending, running toward—was it just a hoax I'd dreamed up so

I didn't go mad? Was it a sign of my own madness: Kari and me running back and forth on the turnpike with our dying girl? I reminded myself that stress can cause doubt and that I had known we would end up there eventually, but I also had a sense that it wasn't time yet and I didn't feel that she was going to go to transplant here. But I was not quite ready to tell Kari about my whispers.

I walked back to the room, where Kari was on the laptop searching for scientific studies. She didn't like what she was finding out about this drug temsirolimus.

"They've used it for adults who have lymphoma, but I couldn't find a study where they used it on children." she said. "The success rate in adults is not impressive. This doesn't feel right, either."

"It doesn't feel right to be here right now to me, either," I said. "I think we imagined that at CHOP they'd have the magic potion that would cure Emily."

"I couldn't live with myself if we enrolled her in that clinical trial and then it made her so sick that she couldn't get the bone marrow transplant. That's our only hope."

She slammed the laptop shut and looked at me with such fear in her face.

"I'm just a mom and these are the best doctors in the world," she said. "Dr. Rheingold told us this is the best thing we can do for Emily right now."

I was just like Kari, with opinions and doubts that were just as strong. I was self-conscious, too. People were going to think we were crazy, racing down here against doctors' orders, and then racing right back to Hershey.

"Let's call Dr. Powell," I said. "We trust him. He's never steered us in the wrong direction. He's not tied to Hershey or to CHOP, so he'll tell us exactly what he thinks."

Dr. Powell didn't pick up, so I laid out the circumstances in a phone message, ending with "Give us your thoughts. It helps us decide."

We sat for a minute in silence. Then Emily spoke.

"I want to go back to Hershey," she said.

"You do? Why?" I asked.

"I like it there better," she said.

"That's three votes out of three," I said. "Kari, go tell the nurses we're going back to Hershey. I'll start packing."

Then Dr. Rheingold came in. She'd heard we were going back to Hershey.

"I really feel the temsirolimus clinical trial offers the best chance to get Emily back into remission," Dr. Rheingold said.

"It just doesn't feel right," I said.

"I wish we had more to offer you here right now," Dr. Rheingold said. "We have some immunotherapy clinical trials for leukemia coming up, one called T cell therapy, that trains your immune cells to fight your cancer."

"I'm very interested in that," said Kari. "I've read a lot about immunotherapy, and it sounds promising."

"I agree," Dr. Rheingold said. "We're ready to start the T cell therapy clinical trial, but we are waiting for approval from the FDA to begin, and it looks like that will be months from now. Emily needs something sooner than that."

"Thanks, Dr. Rheingold," I said. We left CHOP, our hearts heavy, wondering if we had made the right decision.

———————•◦•———————

Once you hit the turnpike on the way to Hershey, you're about an hour away, and I was starting to feel that we had made the right decision. I thought both of them were asleep, but Kari was just faking it until she knew Emily was asleep.

"We're going back because we're comfortable, but really, we're going back there to watch Emily die," Kari whispered.

"No, we're not!" I said. "Not true! Emily's going to make it! I know it."

"You heard what the doctor said," Kari said. She was crying. "Chemo isn't doing anything for Emily and we're going back to Hershey for more chemo."

Kari seemed unnerved that I was not crying, too.

"How are you so calm?" she asked.

"Kari, I had a vision," I said. "I heard a whisper. I've seen it many times, and it's getting stronger each time. I see me walking with Emily. She's weak but she's beaten cancer, and I'm with her at the bone marrow transplant hallway at CHOP, teaching her how to walk again."

"What? Why didn't you tell me this before?" Kari was furious. "Turn the car around right now! We never should have left. We have to go back!"

"Today, we're going back to Hershey," I said. "We don't even have the energy to turn around. This is what we're doing today because that's what Emily wants, and her opinion needs to be heard. It feels to me like the right thing to do now, and we're almost there."

We got off the turnpike exit for Hershey just as Dr. Powell called. He was firm in his advice, telling us we need to get Emily into the temsirolimus clinical trial at CHOP right away.

"We already turned that down," I said. "It didn't feel right to us and we couldn't get hold of you."

"You have to do something right now," Dr. Powell urged.

"Yeah. We know," I said. "Something has to be started soon. We're just arriving at Hershey."

Chapter 12

---·•●•·---

PRAYER REQUESTS

Prayer requests:

—That Emily's blast count goes to ZERO (and stays there forever)

—That Emily continues to feel great—no nausea/vomiting, no pain, no fevers, no infections

—Wisdom for Emily's doctors so they continue to know what to do to cure Emily and the other children here at Hershey

—Strength for all three of us so that we can make it through the next few months

—Kari's journal

February 14, 2012

I had so much pain in my stomach I could barely walk when we entered Hershey, and the reception we got from some of the staff there was chilly. We'd become close to a lot of the nurses and staff in the months we'd lived in that hospital. The staff cared about Emily, and when she wasn't doing well, we felt the sadness and anxiety in the hallways, not just in our room. Upon our return from CHOP, Dr. Lucas didn't want to see us anymore. We never spoke to him again. Our care was transferred to Dr. Moshe Bell, the attending physician who was on service that week.

Kari showed Dr. Bell the clinical trial protocol that Dr. Rheingold had suggested, and overnight Dr. Bell investigated that combination of chemotherapies. He thought this combination, minus the experimental temsirolimus, was a promising alternative. Emily had had three of the four drugs—vincristine, asparaginase, and methotrexate—before and had tolerated them well. He thought it would be a good combination to give Emily. More than that, Dr. Bell's calming manner and the fact that he took the time to research the drugs made it feel right to us. We agreed to go ahead with the chemo.

Emily was happy to be back in Hershey and that made us feel good, too. The fact that one of the chemos, Mitoxantrone, was blue and turned her pee green delighted Emily. She called it the blueberry juice when the nurses would hang it on her IV pole. There were steroids in this chemo cocktail, too, so as they built up in her system, she got moody and very hungry again. However, she did not complain during these weeks. Through it all we admired what a trouper she was. Despite the way this whipsawed her around, she often said she'd do whatever they wanted her to do as long as they controlled her pain. I wondered sometimes if she was hiding some of her pain, just like her parents were trying to do. I saw her reaching for her prayer cloths in her sleep. Kari and I didn't have prayer cloths, but Emily would offer me one when I wasn't feeling well. We had so many loving messages coming from the people reading the blog, which gave us strength and comfort.

As Emily's situation had worsened and our actions became more dramatic, the audience for Kari's blog exploded, and we started a Facebook page for it because it was easier for people to share. Between CaringBridge and Facebook, Kari got hundreds of comments every time she posted.

When I couldn't sleep at night, when I felt too tired to worry, I read messages from our families and our friends and from people we'd never met. The messages of love, the prayers of hope, and the wishes that we would trust in the Lord were often expressed in the same kinds of words. I could read them like chanting in a church: May the Lord be with you....May the Lord watch over Emily....May she feel the healing touch of the Lord. I could read these again and again, and it always soothed my soul when I did. Kari thanked our followers every day for this, always mentioning how Emily asked us to read them to her when she felt low.

In Philipsburg, Big Jim and Pappy Rob set up a bank account to take in the spontaneous donations from the community. Every teller station in every bank branch in Philipsburg, and in the other towns nearby, had that account number taped up on the partition. Churches and community groups, fire stations and schools had started to hold fund-raisers for Emily, and word got out that her favorite color was purple, so people started to wear purple to show their support. Some people dyed their hair purple, and a few guys even dyed their beards purple. That sweet and supportive sentiment started to spread to the schools and church youth groups outside of Philipsburg, and throughout Pennsylvania. Robin would tell story after story of carloads of Girl Scouts who had held a bake sale for Emily bringing their envelope of cash to the bank to deposit, all of them so proud of what they had done, or little boys bringing in all of their birthday money. Stories like these swelled our hearts as we sat in Emily's room, desperate for hope. All we had to do was read comments on Kari's posts and there we would find an outpouring of love and support waiting for us, stronger every day.

We had to take it day by day. We kept asking ourselves if we had made the right decisions. As Kari wrote: "How are we supposed to know what is right when the doctors don't even have all the answers?"

So far, it looks like the chemo is working. Here is her bloodwork over the past week:

Tuesday: White count 115,220; blasts 81%

Wednesday: White count 68,640; blasts 69%

Thursday: White count 16,440; blasts 30%

Friday: White count 6,070; blasts 0%

Saturday: White count 2,150; blasts 0%

Sunday: White count 1,510; blasts 1.9% (although it looks like it went up it probably didn't—the last two counts of 0 blasts were done with a machine which doesn't catch all the blasts and today they looked at it manually and were able to see them)

—Kari's journal

February 12, 2012

They took Emily off steroids on Valentine's Day and she seemed more herself. She was craving cheese balls, and I thought, *Why not? Let's give her whatever she wants because we don't know how long we have.* I went to WalMart and bought a huge tub of those scary neon orange balls, and she wanted to eat them for breakfast. Kari was horrified by this. Her training as a dietitian had caused her a lot of angst since Emily got sick because she knew that indulging in all these poor-quality foods was not helping Emily fight her cancer. She ate so many cheese balls she threw up.

"Mommy was right!" Emily said, smiling, as she dove back into the tub of cheese balls.

Kari did not let up on this. Every time a nurse or a doctor came in to check on Emily, she'd tell the story of Emily's indulgent dad letting her eat whatever she wanted, and how wrong I was. Well, I like to be right, and so does Kari. Now Kari was annoying me, but I wasn't going to send her out of the room. Aunt Kathy arrived, and while they were chatting I found a tiny flying helicopter someone had given Emily. I sent it up flying over Emily's bed, right toward Kari. Emily laughed as I sent it circling around Kari's head, dive-bombing her while she was trying to talk to Aunt Kathy. I missed a turn there and it got tangled up in Kari's hair. As I tried to get the helicopter blades to turn in reverse, it got so deeply tangled in Kari's hair that I had to cut it out of her hair. We thought Aunt Kathy was going to pee herself, she was laughing so hard. This ended up being a good day because we were laughing despite the odds against us.

We needed more of this laughter. We decided we needed to find a way to bring Lucy in for a visit.

As we basically lived in the hospital, Lucy had moved in with my folks, who had even installed a doggie door for her. It was so funny to see Big Jim and Lucy together. Whenever Big Jim took a bite of something, he gave a bite to Lucy. And when he slept in his recliner, he often had Lucy right there on his chest, moving up and down as he breathed, soothed by his snoring. But my dad was not much for visiting the hospital. His back caused him a lot of pain, and long car rides made it worse. Although we couldn't get Big Jim out of Philipsburg often, he made the painful journey to Hershey to bring Lucy to Emily.

While he was making his way through hospital security with the tiny duffel bag that contained Lucy, she started bumping up against the sides of the bag.

"What do you have in there?" one of the guards asked Big Jim.

He grinned, always eager to show off his favorite dog. Big Jim opened the zipper just a little bit, and out popped Lucy's little head. Big Jim grinned. The guards grinned.

"It's my granddaughter's dog," Big Jim said. "She hasn't seen her in weeks, and we all know how much Lucy comforts her."

"I never saw her," said one guard, grinning.

"What dog?" said the other.

The guards directed him to the oncology floor. The whole staff seemed to be in on the "secret" visit. They told Emily there was going to be a big birthday party in the teen lounge on the oncology floor and she was invited. There was no party planned, though. The nurses were so delighted by the idea that a few of them were in the room when Emily opened the door. At first, she was confused, seeing that there were no decorations or cake, or any other guests, but then she saw Big Jim.

When he opened the duffel bag, it was like the first moment Lucy and Emily met. They were nose to nose, exchanging love in that secret language they had. After a few hugs and some tears (from Emily and from Big Jim, Nanny, and Uncle Jim), Lucy immediately took her place on Emily's knees, trying to soothe the pain that she sensed still came from there. Emily had been complaining of stomach pain right before Lucy arrived, but as soon as she saw Lucy, she was smiling and feeling great again. We wished Lucy could be here all the time to smile and cuddle with Emily.

On February 21 we received good news. The test showed the bone marrow was "empty," meaning there were no bad cells there. The chemo was working, but it also killed all her white blood cells, which were at zero. We would have to reassess after her marrow had time to start producing new cells and see if they were healthy cells or blasts.

Then by February 24, we received the discouraging news that the blood work showed 6 percent cancer cells. A more precise test called the MRD (minimal residual disease) test showed Emily had 13 percent blasts in her bone marrow. The doctors were worried that the chemo was not working well enough or even working at all. If the blast cell count was the same or higher at the next bone marrow biopsy in a few days, they would have to try a stronger chemo because the cells were becoming resistant to what they had been using.

We missed THON weekend that February because Emily was too sick to leave the hospital. Some of our THON friends stopped by to visit, which was great for all of us, but it was also sad. The doctors postponed the date for the bone marrow transplant to March 20, hoping the leukemia cells would be less than 1 percent by then. I was full of worry and so was Kari. Could we keep Emily alive for another month when every test showed more cancer in her blood?

There isn't much we can do except wait until the next bone marrow test in two weeks.

Prayers:

1. **That the cancer cells go away—completely.** Typically, most transplant centers will not attempt to do the transplant if there are more than 5% cancer cells left because they know the transplant won't work. That's how important it is that we get this number down.

2. **That Emily is not in pain.** She's been having more pain the past few days and developing some sores that are painful.

3. **That Emily does not develop any infection.** She hasn't run a fever the past few days so it seems the antibiotic she's on is working.

—Kari's journal
February 24, 2012

Even though we had recommitted to Hershey, Kari was still turning the decision over in her mind, and so was I. Before Emily relapsed,

Kari had looked at Emily's chart, where she saw a doctor had noted a chromosomal abnormality. When she researched what she had found, she discovered that the abnormality made it more likely that Emily would be resistant to standard chemotherapy treatments. There wasn't enough research to support changing Emily's treatment, but we had questions as to why we hadn't been told. Kari was reviewing every detail of Emily's treatment, reconsidering every decision we'd made, and reevaluating the advice we followed, and she was starting to feel maybe we should have stayed at CHOP.

"Let's talk with Nurse Karli," Kari said. "She'll have good advice as to what we should do."

We paged Nurse Karli, and when we told her the lab numbers, and about Emily's chromosomal abnormality, she lowered her head as if in prayer before she spoke.

"There's nothing more they can do for you here," she said. "If I were you, I'd take her to CHOP today. It might be her only chance."

I walked out of the room into the hallway because I didn't want Emily to see me upset. I steadied myself against the wall and conjured up that vision of her and me in the bone marrow transplant hallway at CHOP. It was not a whisper—I didn't hear it—but I summoned it to support me. I saw it vividly in my mind. That was where we were going, I decided.

I felt a hand on my shoulder that interrupted my vision. It was Dr. John Neely.

"Can you and Kari join me in the consultation room?" he asked gently. "The blasts are increasing. We need to make a plan for what's next."

At the table, Dr. Neely was blunt.

"It's time to set up hospice care for Emily," he said. "We don't have any more tools to treat her cancer. We'll treat her with chemo one more time to slow the blasts growing, but they'll be back. You need to take her home and enjoy the days you have left with her."

Kari started to cry. I felt the anguish, too, but I didn't believe the doctor so I didn't cry. I was strengthened by my vision of the walk in the hallway.

"We're not going home and we're not going to hospice. We're going to CHOP. I'm paging Dr. Rheingold."

Dr. Rheingold called me back from her home. I could hear her children in the background.

"We need help," I said. "Emily's cancer is growing again, and the doctors say it's time for hospice. Is the clinical trial using temsirolimus still open to Emily?"

"Unfortunately, that trial is no longer an option. The chemotherapy that Emily just got at Hershey disqualified her for that trial," Dr. Rheingold said. "But this is amazing that you paged me today, because the FDA just gave us approval to try T cell therapy on pediatric patients. It was the last email that I read before I left work, and the approval came much sooner than expected. I think Emily will qualify for that trial."

I grabbed Kari's hand and squeezed it hard as I put Dr. Rheingold on speakerphone.

"You mean that the T cell therapy clinical trial has just opened for children and CHOP is ready to enroll patients?" I asked, grinning at Kari.

"Yes," said Dr. Rheingold. "Emily could be the first."

Kari was looking at me, eyes full of grateful disbelief.

"We're coming," I said. "You have her full care as soon as we get there."

"See you soon," Dr. Rheingold said.

For the first time in a long while, we had hope. Kari had, in her way, been following her whispers. Over the months since Dr. Rheingold had described how CHOP was preparing to run the T cell therapy clinical trial, Kari had not been able to get the idea out of her mind. She had spent hours searching for places where it had been tried, and trying to understand the science behind the treatment. She had read all about how T cells could be genetically modified to attack cancer. This singular focus was her form of the whispers. She had been drawn to this method repeatedly in her research. And me, I had my vision of Emily and me in the bone marrow transplant hallway at CHOP that I had tended to so carefully. It now seemed to be coming true.

As we walked out of the pediatric cancer unit at Hershey that last time, the corridor was lined with our beloved nurses and other medical staff who had been through so much with us in the last several months. I think we were leaving just as the shift was changing because there seemed to be more people in the hallway than we normally saw on the floor, and many of them were crying. Some of them were trying to hide it, but some of them weren't. That was hard.

There was so much we wanted to say to them, so much gratitude we had for them. Also, I wanted to tell them not to cry. We had hope. Emily was going to beat this thing. Maybe if I had said that to them they would have told me no, they'd seen this movie before, and it didn't end well. And I wanted to say to them that Emily was not like those other patients. I wanted to tell them that she was going to live and that it would be unlike anything that had ever been seen or done before. Emily had the whole world pulling for her, writing to her, and praying for her, I wanted to say, and she was going to survive.

Chapter 13

---•-•●•-•---

THE TROJAN HORSE
AND THE CHIMERA

lthough we knew T cell therapy was our last chance to save Emily, we didn't feel a sense of doom. My hopes and prayers and Kari's faith in science, as well as the prayers of thousands of people we'd never met, had converged to bring us this miracle. I had never given up hope that something would arrive to save Emily, while Kari's form of faith was her focus on this T cell therapy. When we'd come to CHOP that second time, just a few weeks ago, Dr. Rheingold had told us they were ready for the T cell therapy clinical trial, but the approval was still months away, much too far off in the distance to be of any help to Emily.

Then suddenly, it had seemed when there was no other place to turn, it was ready.

As crazy as we had seemed, rushing from one hospital to the other, driven by visions and worries, shouting at an officer on the highway, praying, screaming, pacing, crying—there had been something driving Kari and me to the best solution. Whatever it was that brought us to CHOP on that March evening, we knew Emily still had a chance, and that was all that mattered.

The next morning, Dr. Stephan Grupp, the pediatric oncologist in charge of this clinical trial, and his research team came into Emily's room. They explained the clinical trial and answered our questions. I liked Dr. Grupp instantly. He's tall and affable, the kind of guy who looks at you directly. We instantly trusted his mix of spirit and seriousness. He felt solid and calm. I knew he would not sugarcoat the risks of enrolling Emily in this trial. His having his team with him to answer any and all questions impressed me.

"I'm not here to sell you on this treatment," he said. "If anything I say makes you uncomfortable, question me. Think hard about whether you want Emily involved in this clinical trial. It offers no guarantees."

Dr. Grupp, head of the hospital's immunotherapy research and transplant program, described himself modestly as the general contractor for T cell therapy. He was a brilliant scientist, an expert in stem cell transplants, leading the big team of lab technicians, researchers, nurses, and doctors dedicated to saving Emily. He was the person who Dr. Carl June, the scientist who had created the T cell therapy, chose to run the pediatric trial.

To begin, they would harvest Emily's T cells—a type of white blood cell that helps fight infection—in a process called apheresis. Then, in the lab, they would genetically modify them, reprogramming the cells to enable them to identify cancer cells and kill them. If it worked, it could eliminate her cancer. Dr. Grupp continued to emphasize the *if.*

"We have only treated three patients in the world with this," he said. "Two of them went into remission and remain there. None of them had the same type of leukemia as your daughter. None of them are children; they were men in their sixties. We know very, very little. There is a very big chance it will not work."

"Is it going to make her sick?" I asked. I didn't want her to suffer. That was the main thing. I knew Kari felt the same way. We could not wish on her any more suffering unless it led to a cure.

"This is not toxic like chemo. We're using her own immune cells to fight her disease," he said. "There may be significant toxicities, which could be life threatening, but not the same as those posed by chemo. It's likely that she'll feel like she's had the worst case of the flu in the world. There could be other things that we aren't expecting. It is hard to know what to expect when so few people have ever received this treatment."

"How long will treatment take?" I asked.

"We don't know," he said.

"If it does work, how long will it last?" Kari asked.

"We don't know," Dr. Grupp said.

"After it works, will Emily need a bone marrow transplant?" Kari asked.

"We don't know," Dr. Grupp replied. "There's so much we don't know because Emily will be the first child in the world treated this way. We want to increase knowledge, and we want to move the medical ball forward, and we want to help kids in the future. Those are the big-picture goals. But our immediate focus is to cure Emily, and we'll work as hard as we can to do that."

———— ··◦·· ————

We signed the consent forms to begin treatment, a six-week process that would start the next day when a catheter would be surgically placed into a vein in Emily's neck. The following day, the apheresis machine would be connected to the catheter to collect Emily's blood. We watched through the window at the top of the machine as a centrifuge spun her blood around to separate out her T cells, returning the rest of the blood to her once the cells had been harvested. The centrifuge works like the spin cycle on a washing machine. We watched the technician adjust the speed of the spin to collect as many T cells as possible. For every liter of blood they collected from Emily they harvested a billion cells into a bag that hung on the side of the machine. They took that bag of cells to the lab immediately to begin the process of genetically modifying them so they would be able to attack cancer cells. In mid-April, the reprogrammed cells would be infused back into her, revved up for the fight. Emily would get the cells in three infusions: Day 1, 10 percent; Day 2, 30 percent; and Day 3, 60 percent. If all went well, the infusions would be done on an outpatient basis.

Emily wasn't paying much attention to what we were about to do. At that moment, she was feeling well and resigned to whatever next thing people were going to do to her body. Her attitude had become practical. This had been her life for nearly two years, and she'd become used to it. She rarely complained unless she was in pain. The doctors treated her pain with a fentanyl patch, leaving her alert without the effects of the morphine, and brighter because she was not in pain.

We had six weeks to wait. We kept Emily busy during the long days in the hospital by reading books. More arrived every day, sometimes several at a time. When we were at Hershey waiting for the bone marrow transplant, Kari had created a plan to keep Emily entertained for those weeks we would be quarantined with her after they gave her the donor cells. Kari had invited people to send Emily books, and we were astonished by the response. We got books from all over the country, and even from other countries. We got new books and used books that had been cherished by children who had outgrown them, and the cards that came were filled with love and prayers. When Emily was out of sorts, or in pain, the easiest way to settle her down was to allow her to choose from the bottomless box of books. She could read as many as she liked, and there were always more. It was a blessing bigger than any of the people who sent them would ever know.

On an unseasonably warm March day, we convinced the staff to give us a day pass out of the hospital so Emily could get some sunlight and fresh air. Robin and Pam were there. We got the pass right after Emily finished giving Robin another art lesson. The nurses were all business when they told us we could go out for six hours and six hours only, cautioning us to be very careful to protect Emily from germs.

We took Emily to a park nearby, and Kari and I hovered near her as she moved around the play structure, frantic that she not slip and fall, break a bone. Kari covered Emily's hands with sanitizer and wanted to reapply it every five minutes. I think she would have wiped down the whole play structure if she could have gotten over the embarrassment that would have produced. We were sticking so close by Emily that we heard her introducing herself to the other kids on the playground. She was matter-of-fact about how she had cancer, explaining that was why she had no hair, but she was getting treated and she would be getting better soon. The kids were great. They took it all at face value, never teasing her, just including her as she was.

Emily said she wanted us to leave her alone to play pirates with her new friends. She endured more warnings and admonitions from me and Kari that she be careful, and one more application of hand sanitizer before we stepped away. Just as we turned to sit on the bench with Robin and Pam, we heard Emily yell out to the other kids, "Follow me!" And then we heard that sound, like the ping of a baseball hitting an aluminum bat, and turned around to see Emily flat on her back. She hadn't seen the monkey bars in the glare of the harsh winter sun and had run full force into them. She had a purple lump on her forehead about the size of half a golf ball, and it was growing. Things started to move in slow motion.

I gathered her up and sprinted to the car with Kari, Robin, and Pam jogging behind. Kari was yelling frantically, "Tom, you have to run faster!" I laid Emily out on the passenger seat while everyone else piled in the back. We were all frantic, each of us convinced that we were the one who could have, should have, stopped her.

We didn't know Philadelphia very well. Kari was shouting out directions back to the hospital from the GPS.

I remembered the way back, but it didn't align with the GPS directions. I went to turn when Kari emphatically yelled, "You are going the wrong way!" I believed that I was entering the correct on-ramp so I took it anyway. The GPS updated, and then everyone calmed down because we knew we were on the fastest route back. Kari was terrified Emily's blood wouldn't clot and we'd lose her from bleeding on the brain, not leukemia. I wasn't thinking about bleeding. I was thinking about permanent brain damage. Fortunately, Emily sustained no damage, except for a big knot on her forehead. That black and blue knot made me wince every time I focused on it, but it did not faze Emily.

The days dragged on in the hospital as we waited for the T cells to be ready. In the meantime, Emily received what we hoped to be her very last round of chemotherapy to keep the leukemia from growing out of control. It was an intense five-day combination of chemotherapy drugs—Cytoxan, etoposide, and clofarabine—which made her very ill. We were used to her being nauseous from the chemo, but this time the nausea and vomiting was much worse. After a few weeks she had lost so much weight she needed a nasogastric (NG) tube, a long, thin flexible tube that delivered nutrients directly into the stomach. Her skin looked gray and was very sensitive. Her skin ripped every time the nurses changed the dressing on her port. She received daily blood and platelet transfusions.

It was a lonely time for me and Kari. Emily was confined to her room for the most part, so she wasn't exposed to germs, and the confinement made us cranky. We did have a few family members visit, but we were always worried they would bring a cold or other illness into the room.

Prayers needed:
1) That Emily no longer suffers from nausea/vomiting
2) That this chemo regimen puts her in a solid remission so she doesn't have to go through any other treatments before transplant
3) That she doesn't get any infections while her counts are low
4) That she remains brave and strong

—Kari's journal
March 11, 2012

While we waited for the T cells to be ready, Kari continued to learn as much as she could about T cell therapy. There wasn't much online about the treatment, but there was some information about Dr. Carl June, the brilliant researcher at Penn Medicine, who had devised this inventive method for using HIV as a vehicle to treat cancer. At CHOP we were surrounded by scientists at the forefront of this incredible idea, so, as we got to know more about the treatment, we got to know more about the people involved in the research.

We learned that the navy had put Dr. June through medical school during the Vietnam War, funding his research into bone marrow transplantation with a focus on treating people who had been irradiated in a nuclear disaster, the military's big concern during the Cold War. After the Cold War ended, the military assigned Dr. June to AIDS research, specifically the T cells damaged by HIV. Working with T cells deepened his understanding of the immune system. When his wife, Cindy, died of cancer, Dr. June decided to honor her by focusing all his energy on the cure for cancer. He wanted to combine what he had learned about the immune system through his HIV research and what he knew about cell propagation through the study of bone marrow transplantation. Most doctors study either cancer or the immune system, but he had studied both and could look at cancer in a novel way. Everything in his past had prepared him for this moment. Every experience lent something.

When Dr. June and his colleague, Dr. Bruce Levine, began studying how the body fights disease, researchers had been making progress, but very slow progress, in pursuit of training the immune system to attack cancer. The body's immune system has a sophisticated response to disease, able to annihilate a wide array of threats. When pathogens assault the body, white blood cells identify the invaders quickly and react with a multi-pronged assault, but the system doesn't respond to cancer. The immune system is trained to distinguish between self and non-self, meaning that if the system is working properly, it will not attack its own cells. Cancer cells are mutated cells that originate in the body. This is why the immune system does not identify them as a threat, and cancer can grow unchecked.

Still, the promise of training the body to defend itself from cancer, and to not have to bombard patients with chemotherapy or radiation that kills both cancer cells and healthy cells, was such an elegant idea that it sparked the imaginations of scientists for decades.

Researchers identified many kinds of white blood cells and the chemical networks involved in keeping us disease free. The main actors include B cells, T cells, and Dendritic Cells (DC). The DC and the B cells are scouts, first to recognize and shine a light on the invaders. DC's vacuum up the invaders and signal the T cells to respond. T cells, as captains of the immune system, direct and activate the responses of other T cells and B cells. B cells, armed with antibodies that lock onto the surface, neutralize the invaders. Once researchers had a better understanding of how the various players of the immune system responded, the goal became making the T cell a more effective captain in identifying and attacking cancer.

Researchers figured out how to harvest the T cells from the patient's blood by separating them out in a specifically designed centrifuge, the one Emily had been hooked up to. Then they developed techniques for how to grow T cells in a lab by the billions, how to characterize these cells, and how to prepare them for reinfusion, thereby vastly increasing their presence in the bloodstream.

Once they had T cells, and lots of them, the next huge advancement was when they genetically engineered a synthetic molecule that could be attached to the T cells, giving them the ability to recognize and destroy cancer cells. These synthetic immune cells are called CAR T cells, with "CAR" standing for Chimeric Antigen Receptors. The CAR on the outside of a T cell is composed of an antibody that, like the naturally occurring B cell antibody, binds to the cancer antigen. The big difference from a naturally occurring antibody is that a CAR has a portion that is embedded in the cell membrane through to the inside of the cell (the cytoplasm), signaling the T cell to attack the cancer. Amazing! The problem in the early versions of CAR T cells is that they got exhausted rapidly. Not enough of them stuck around long enough to make the cancer disappear. As effective as CAR T cells were in the lab and in mice, still more work needed to be done to make the human immune system capable of knocking out cancer.

This is where June and Levine's experience with HIV advanced cancer therapy. Dr. June had studied how the HIV uses the T cell as a host. It breaks through the T cell membrane and takes over, slipping its genes into the T cell chromosomes, so the T cell produces the virus that in turn destroys it and other T cells. Dr. June figured out how to combine cutting edge technologies and apply these to help cancer patients. First, he knew that researchers had shown that it was possible to take out the genes that made HIV a killer and use its powerful delivery mechanism to place the gene for the cancer-killing CAR inside that modified T cell. The disabled HIV delivers the gene that scientists designed, but it could never cause HIV disease in the patient. Dr. Levine brought all his experience in engineering T cells to growing them in a clean room laboratory with microscopic beads that produced billions of CAR T cells. When these specially modified cells were infused into a patient with cancer, the cancer-killing CAR T cell continued to replicate inside the body, thereby creating a living cancer killing drug that could stay on the job until the cancer was completely gone.

Dr. June compares the disabled HIV delivering the CAR gene to the Trojan horse from Greek history. The Greeks were losing a ten-year war against the Trojans when they came up with the idea for a sneak attack. The Greeks pretended to surrender and left a tribute for the Trojans in the form of a huge wooden horse, with a note announcing their withdrawal and defeat. The Trojans wheeled the big horse inside the walls of the city and started celebrating when suddenly a trap door opened in the horse's belly and out popped the Greek special forces, who won the battle. This would be Dr. June's brilliant sneak-attack to put the gene for the CAR hidden in the belly of the disabled HIV that would create the CAR T cell that would slay the cancer.

As Dr. June described it to me later, "When the CAR T cells are injected, they act like supercharged killers on steroids. The Trojan horse of the HIV slips through the cells' defenses and heads straight to the tumor, where those chimeric cells divide, quickly numbering hundreds of millions of cells specifically programmed to destroy the cancer."

What a fantastic idea, this hybrid serial killer of cancer. Just one CAR T cell can kill 1,000 tumor cells. Yes, that's right: a ratio of 1-to-1,000. There is no precedent for this in cancer medicine. With every other medicine, you ingest it, metabolize it, and then take another dose. CAR–T cell therapy is the first living drug, capable of regenerating in the body for years.

————··●··————

During that six-week wait for the T cells to be reprogrammed, we had to be careful not to expose Emily to germs because if she got an infection it might delay her participation in the clinical trial. We washed our hands carefully every time we entered her room and wiped down any item that came in, lest it carry germs to Emily. As the day of the infusion approached, we were relieved we'd succeeded in keeping her safe.

The week before getting her CAR–T cell infusion, the hospital was buzzing about Emily. If this worked, Emily and the doctors involved in the treatment would make medical history. The nurses and the doctors were excited.

The CHOP public relations department wanted to film the moment when Emily got her CAR T cells. They asked us if we'd be willing to be interviewed on that day, and if Emily might participate, too. We needed to talk this over as a family, and I was all for it. Six weeks before, the doctors were telling us to set up hospice so we could say goodbye to our little girl, but here we were. We were not just in a holding pattern anymore, not just surviving. I wanted the whole world to witness this moment of hope. Kari hesitated, though.

"We've spent six weeks keeping her infection free and now they want to bring in a bunch of people and cameras?" Kari asked. "I don't think that's a very good idea."

"Emily's going to change the world," I said. "I think it's great that the hospital wants to record this moment for history."

"I don't know, Tom," Kari said. "This is all so delicate. Things can still go wrong. Why should we introduce anything that might put Emily at risk?"

"What if I work with the hospital to make it as safe as possible for her?" I said. "If they can protect her, would that make it okay?"

"Maybe," Kari said.

CHOP did work with us to make Emily safe. On Tuesday, April 17, they set up a separate hospital room for us to do the interview and made sure it, and the crew and their equipment, was carefully sanitized before filming began. The cameras were all set up when we walked in. Emily sat down on the bed with her head angled into her chest, uninterested in this spectacle. She didn't want to perform in front of a bunch of strangers with cameras. When the interviewer asked her what was going to happen to her that day, she looked up at him and then looked away without saying a word.

"They are going to take away your cancer, right Emily?" I said, prompting her to respond. I think she just wanted to get on with it.

"They're going to take my cancer away," she said softly, without much conviction.

When the interview was over, Dr. Grupp himself attached the syringe full of CAR T cells to her port. But just before he started the infusion, Emily called a halt to it. The preservative for the cells had a horrible stinky odor of creamed corn and Emily didn't want the infusion to go any further until she had a popsicle to cover up that taste. Dr. Grupp obliged, and then we watched as he pushed in the syringe full of an army of cells ready to attack Emily's cancer. We had so much hope riding on these cells.

After the cells were in and Dr. Grupp left, I pulled a chair up to Emily's head so I could touch her as I talked to her. I felt the hopes of all the people online who had been praying that day. Just to look at the comments on the blog was to hear a mighty chorus of praise, of well wishes and incantations of joy. I wanted to transmit that feeling I felt from the world directly into my girl's exhaustion and confusion. How would Nurse Karli describe this? I couldn't draw pictures like she did.

"When they took all that blood from you, they did it because they're building an army," I said. "They're training the army to fight your cancer, Emily's army, and it's going to be awesome how powerful that army is."

She was sleepy, but her eyes were open and she was listening intently.

"They took some of your cells, the ones that fight infections, and made them super strong and focused on one job and one job only: to fight your cancer," I explained. "And you're going to fight, too. This medicine the doctors made is just for you. You're going to have to stay strong while it works fighting your cancer. How hard are you going to fight?"

"I'll fight as hard as I can, Daddy," she said.

I think they kind of overdid it on the premedications for that first injection. She was on antinausea medications, Benadryl, and morphine, which made her loopy. After the infusion she kept asking us when she was going to get her T cells. Emily had tolerated the first injection of 10 percent of the cells so well they told us that we didn't have to stay in the hospital overnight. She was exhausted from the procedure, though. She fell asleep in the car on the way to Kari's sister Kristen's, who lives thirty minutes away in Delaware, and she didn't wake up until the next morning, sleeping seventeen hours in all. This gave Kari time to describe

Emily's T cell therapy infusion on the blog, and our support network checked the blog several times a day to reassure themselves and to leave us comments.

> The first thing I do when I wake up in the morning is check to make sure that Emily made it through the night. Then I have my coffee and say my prayers for Emily.
> —Nikki Lash.

> I can't stop thinking about her. My heart goes out to Em and her family. My daughter Hailey is 13 and she has been following Emily's page with me. She is doing a video for her and also asked at youth group this evening if they could all say a prayer for Emily and they did. Praying every time I think of her, which is pretty much 24/7. God bless you all.
> —Andrea Jean Hill

Although Kari and I were involved in the day-to-day care of Emily, we had not lost sight of the fact that she could be making medical history, and people who had loved ones who suffered through cancer brought those emotions to Emily's story. There was a lot riding on the shoulders of one little girl.

Emily received 30 percent of the cells on the second day of infusion. After Emily got that second infusion, we had a fun night at Kristen's. Becky and Ariana came to visit, and I loved watching them washing Becky's car, spraying each other with the hose. It was like the times before Emily's relapse. Kari filmed me giving Emily a horsey ride, her on my back and me bucking around Kristen's living room. That night she spiked a fever, so we took her to the ER. Dr. Grupp had predicted this might happen, as it had happened to the adult patients. By the time we got her to the ER, her temperature had returned to normal, but they admitted her anyway just to be safe. That morning she got the final injection of the remaining 60 percent of the T cells, and that afternoon she spiked a fever again, but this time is was much higher: 104.9.

The doctors said not to worry about the fever too much. Children can tolerate a pretty high fever, and she was in the best place possible for someone who was sick. But she was getting worse. Over Friday and Saturday, she was constantly vomiting, and we had to plead with her to try to keep swallowing Tylenol for the fever. But she would throw up almost everything she swallowed, so the Tylenol wasn't doing much good. Her fever climbed to 106 degrees and she complained of her entire body being painful.

On Sunday her blood pressure started dropping and she became lethargic and confused. Every time she breathed in and out, she would moan and grunt, her little body working hard to breathe. Her fever remained between 104 and 106, and she woke up in the middle of the night describing a pond in her room, and at one point that night she thought she had Lucy in the bed with her. The doctors ordered antibiotics because they thought this was an infection, but that didn't make any sense to us. We thought she was reacting to the T cells, that maybe they had already started to work even though in the older men it had taken ten days, not two, to develop symptoms. No one knew what was happening for sure and the antibiotics did not seem to be working. Kari and I started to panic.

The PICU staff came in to evaluate Emily and took her right away. They rolled her bed directly into the PICU. Kari only had enough time to post a brief message to Emily's supporters on the blog.

> Em not good. Breathing not good. Blood pressure and oxygen low. Pain. Transferring to ICU. They think it's an inflammatory response to the T cells. Also final bone marrow showed 62 percent blasts.
>
> —Kari's journal
> April 22, 2012

We had no idea how much Emily was going to suffer over the next few days or the horrible decisions we were going to face.

Chapter 14

SAY GOODBYE TO EMILY

Emily came into the PICU confused and in pain. She was sobbing and scared of her new surroundings. We noticed that she was struggling to breathe, and her breath sounded raspy. We could feel the urgency of the medical staff as they infused her with IV fluids and medications, monitoring her blood pressure and heart rate. It wasn't long before the PICU attending physician, Dr. Alexis Topjian, pulled us out into the hallway. We could sense the seriousness of the moment in her bright and warm brown eyes.

"Your little girl is very sick," Dr. Topjian said. "Her kidneys are shutting down. She's struggling to breathe, and her heart rate is incredibly high. She's dehydrated and her blood pressure is dropping. We're going to give her fluids and several blood products. And we have to talk about putting her on a ventilator. Her oxygen level is low, and she's working very hard to breathe. She's in acute respiratory distress."

"Do you really think she needs a ventilator?" asked Kari.

"Yes, that's what I recommend. The ventilator will breathe for Emily so her body doesn't have to work as hard," she explained.

"Then I think the ventilator is the best decision," I said.

"We'll put her on the lightest form of support," Dr. Topjian said. "She'll need to be sedated, put into a medically induced coma, to endure the ventilator. We'll keep an eye on how she responds to these fluids. We call this the stepwise approach. We give her a little bit and see how she responds. Then maybe we hold off, or maybe we give her a little more. You're going to see a lot of me in the next few hours. I'll be spending a lot of time in Emily's room."

"Thank you, Doctor," I said. "Thanks for taking such good care of Emily."

"We're doing the best we can," Dr. Topjian said. "You might want to say a few words to her now, explain to her what we're about to do."

By this time Emily was groggy and I'm not sure how much she heard of what I was saying. Kari and I believed she got the sense of the love that was coming to her from the touch of my hand.

"Emily, the doctor thinks you're working too hard to breathe and they're going to give you medicine to help with that," I said. "They're going to put you on a machine to help you breathe, and they'll have to put you to sleep for that. Do you understand me?"

Emily nodded her head yes, and when I glanced over at Kari, I could see the tears welling in the corners of her eyes.

"We may not be able to talk to you for a while, so we wanted you to remember how much we love you, how much we are fighting for you. So are all the doctors and nurses here," I said. "All the people who have been reading your story online are praying for you. Are you strong enough to keep fighting?"

For the first time in almost two years of fighting cancer, she shook her head no.

"You've got to pray, Emily," I said. I understood her wanting to give up, but she couldn't, not when we were so close to her getting well. "Pray for the strength to get through the night and to keep fighting. Trust your dad about this. You are going to beat it."

I saw a little nod of her head: yes.

"Stay with me, Daddy," she said softly.

"I will," I said. "I'll be right by your side."

She faintly gripped my hand. I felt like our entire lives would end if this was the last time I would ever talk to her.

A swarm of nurses and doctors entered the room to sedate her. They put a breathing tube into Emily's airway and attached the ventilator. They also inserted an arterial line to monitor her blood pressure and a femoral line, another central line for all her medications, one with three ports. With all the medications and fluids and the ventilator, she stabilized and even got better for a few hours, but then she got much worse.

As she'd predicted, Dr. Topjian was in Emily's room most of the night. At one point she took her focus off the machines and turned it on us.

"Maybe you two need a break from this," Dr. Topjian said. "Most parents do. They stay in the waiting room because it can get hard to be here."

"I can't go," I said. "I promised Emily I'd never leave her."

Dr. Topjian understood how seriously I took that promise.

That's how it was that night. I sat next to Emily, holding her hand, wearing a surgical gown and mask, as the doctor ordered. Kari sat at the foot of Emily's bed and Dr. Topjian moved among various machines, scanning the numbers and adjusting the levels of the medications and fluids they were giving Emily to keep her alive. Dr. Topjian's focus was as deep as her compassion. I was amazed how she chose to live this life of brinksmanship, able to concentrate when a life hung in the balance.

Although we'd known her for only a few hours, we were completely comfortable with her in charge. She treated us as part of a team, not to be talked down to, as if, even though she was the medical expert, this was a problem we would address together.

Again Dr. Topjian called us out into the hallway.

"Her lungs are filling with fluid," Dr. Topjian said.

"Well, then should you give her less IV fluids?" I asked.

"When your body is really inflamed, as hers is, fluid leaks out of your blood vessels into your tissues," Dr Topjian said. "Although her body, her tissues, are filled with fluid, it's not in her blood vessels, which is why her kidneys are failing. Her lungs are getting worse. I've talked to Dr. Grupp and we agreed that to reduce the inflammation there, we have to consider administering steroids."

"She's been on steroids many times," Kari said.

"We don't have a lot of information on this, but we know that steroids can pose a risk to her CAR T cells," Dr. Topjian said. "They can kill those cells, so there may be a tough decision up ahead."

"We can't give her anything that will kill the CAR T cells!" Kari said.

"That doesn't sound like a good idea," I agreed.

"It's a risk you have to consider," Dr. Topjian said. "If she can't breathe, those cells won't do her any good. The goal is to keep her alive so those cells can fight her cancer."

Dr. Topjian excused herself. Kari and I stood in the hallway, unable to make this enormous decision.

"What do we do?" Kari said. "We give her steroids to save her life, which could kill the CAR T cells. Then she'll suffer until the cancer takes her? Or do we not give her steroids and just keep going so that we can keep the CAR T cells?"

"I don't know," I said. "I just…I'm trying so hard to feel what's best, to feel what's right, but I'm not feeling anything."

I tried calling Dr. Grupp, but he didn't respond. Then I realized it was two in the morning.

I went to the hospital atrium and called Dr. Powell. He was at home in bed but he answered. I described Emily's dismal vital signs. He recommended giving the steroids and mentioned that it takes steroids some time to work and that the odds of Emily surviving this were already not good. I returned to Emily's room.

"I don't know what we should do," Kari said. "But if we don't stop whatever it is that is happening, we might lose her."

"I don't know. I want to think about it."

"I know that. But we don't have much time."

This was the cycle that we went through every few hours: Dr. Topjian would give Emily fluids and medications; her blood pressure would stabilize, and we'd relax a bit, thinking that she was doing okay. Then her oxygen and blood pressure would start to drop more.

The next morning, as her vital signs fluctuated in a lethal range, everything looked so grim. Her lungs were still filling with fluid, so we agreed to the steroids, but they didn't seem to have much effect. She was getting sicker, and then Dr. Topjian had to go home. She'd been supervising Emily's care for eighteen hours and it was time for her to get some rest. We were so sad to see her go. It wasn't that we distrusted the next doctor—not at all. It was that we had grown to admire Dr. Topjian so much, to trust her so completely. She had kept Emily alive through that difficult night and we couldn't picture being in Emily's room without her calm and competent presence to keep us steady.

I thought of the little girl who came into Dr. Topjian's care eighteen hours earlier, confused and sad, but awake, and with us in this fight. After Dr. Topjian left, the doctors decided to switch Emily to a more powerful ventilator called an oscillating ventilator, a monster of a thing that made a huge thunking sound like an unbalanced washing machine. Plus, they added a third medication to support her blood pressure. I was sitting next to her bed holding her hand, looking at the monitors, and I was thinking, *I don't understand how this happens. How does she leave us? Is her blood pressure going to go to zero? Does her heart just stop?* I wanted to ask those questions, but I didn't want to hear the answers.

"Tom, we need to prepare ourselves for the fact that Emily might die," Kari said. "I don't have the kind of faith you have."

"She's going to make it," I said.

"I believe in God, but I look at the science part of this," Kari said. "All the signs point to her not making it much longer, and we need to prepare for that."

"When the doctors saw me talking to Emily, one of them told me that she had so much anesthesia in her that she had no idea what I was saying," I said. "But then she would nod her head and acknowledge my questions. I know Emily is still there. She's still fighting. We can't give up hope."

"I'm not hopeless, Tom," Kari said. "But we have to be realistic."

When Dr. Robert Berg took over from Dr. Topjian, he motioned us into the hallway to talk.

"I'm looking at Emily's numbers, and by every measurement she's steadily declining," he said. "I would say she has only a one-in-one-thousand chance of making it through the night. It's time to call your families to prepare them. It's time for them to come to say goodbye to Emily."

Chapter 15

———··●··———

WE BELIEVE

Em was in too much respiratory distress and low BP. They had to intubate her. She is on a ventilator and sedated so she is not aware of what is going on. Had to administer steroids to stabilize her and save her life, but steroids kill T cells. They will check her bone marrow today to see if T cells had a chance to kill any leukemia and see if any T cells are still there. Will be on ventilator for several days, maybe up to a week.

—Kari's journal

April 23, 2012

Emily had two IV poles holding seventeen medication pumps, with wires and tubes connected everywhere on her fragile body. We wanted to lie beside her to provide comfort, but we couldn't get around all the tubes and wires. She was retaining so much fluid that she was swollen almost beyond recognition. The ventilator shook her body with such a strong vibration that it had worn through the skin at the back of her throat. Blood was bubbling out of her mouth and running down her cheeks. I wanted to wipe it off her face, but I was scared to touch her. The nurse came in to check her vitals and dabbed a bit of it away.

"I can take a lot," I said to the nurse, "but I can't take looking at her that way. Is it okay for me to wipe off the blood?"

"You can't wipe it off," the nurse said. "Her platelets are low and that liquid around her mouth is how she's clotting. If you wipe it off, she'll bleed to death."

You know how people talk about hell on earth? That's what that room felt like to me and Kari.

———————••●••———————

My mom was already at the hospital with us, so she knew the dire condition Emily was in, and Kari's mom, dad, step-mom, Sharon, and aunt Kathy were on their way. I knew Aunt Laurie was coming, too. She had a few days off from her residency rotation at Hershey and had planned her visit long before this crisis. I was glad she was coming, as she and Kari loved to discuss science.

I called my brothers, Jim and Greg, who said they would come right away and bring Aunt Sally along with them. I asked them to hold off a minute while I called Becky and Ariana. Maybe they could all come together on that long drive. The girls decided to drop everything and come, even though it was finals week at Penn State.

Becky picked up Ariana and two other members of THON, who met up with my brothers. Kari's sisters Kristen and Brenda were coming, too. Even her youngest sister, Lindsey, would be there, though she was eight and a half months pregnant. She wanted to see Emily so badly and she feared she'd never get another chance once the baby came. There were going to be a lot of our family members gathered in that waiting room.

Kari and I were complementary opposites, but for the first time since Emily got sick, we were not on the same page. Before this moment, our jobs of hope and science had never been in conflict, both contributing to the same goal: getting Emily to her cure. Kari had no more hope and she felt that trying to raise it was a waste of energy. She sat dumbstruck with grief, unable to leave the room, holding Emily's feet and massaging them because she didn't want them to be cold. She had a playlist of Emily's favorite music on her phone, which she had positioned near Emily's head in the hope that those tunes she loved could cover over the *BANG, BANG, BANG* sound of the ventilator, but they didn't, at least not for anyone else in the room.

Kari wanted the room to be peaceful so Emily could rest, using what energy she had to stay alive. She wanted it to be just her and me in the room with Emily most of the time. She had taken out the prayer cloths my mother brought Emily and set up many of the religious tokens the followers of the blog sent us. We needed anything and everything to get through this. Kari thought it was only a matter of time.

I thought the opposite. I knew that Emily was in there fighting as hard as any human could fight to stay alive. I figured a little six-year-old girl needed reinforcements to keep going when her body was making it so tough. I wanted to bring the energy of the world into that room to support her, the energy not just from me and Kari, but from all the members of our family who loved her so much and had been there with us during these years of struggle. They all needed to bring that to her, along with the avalanche of positive feelings I knew were coming from the thousands of people all over the country and all over the world who were keeping Emily in their thoughts and prayers. Right then I couldn't spend time on the blog reading those prayers, but I knew that they were there. And when I'd sit with Emily and touch the part of her hand or her arm that was not covered with wires and tubes, I'd shut my eyes and imagine all those fingers on keyboards and cell phones sending their wishes for healing and for life through my hand to my struggling little girl. I wanted all of that love to come into the room to speak to her.

Emily was going to pull through this. It was only a matter of time, and we had to hold that hope for her, and reinforce that energy so that she felt it, too. I knew she could hear us even though she was in a coma. The feeling of that love and the sound of those words, I believed, would give her a reason to fight to stay in our world. I believed she would hear these voices and hold on.

My mom had gone in to pray over Emily while I was out in the hallway calling people. She was carrying a message from Lucy, too. Big Jim was in too much back pain to travel, so he stayed home with Lucy. When my mom called him to tell him that Emily's odds were now at 1-in-1,000, he said he knew something was up because Lucy told him. Just at the moment when we were getting that bad news, it seemed, Lucy's left ear folded down like it had collapsed, and it had stayed that way. Lucy was so connected to Emily that she sensed this crisis even though she was 250 miles away. That ear was still folded down, and knowing what it meant caused Big Jim to dissolve into tears.

"You tell Emily about Lucy," he told my mom. "You tell her that Lucy is pulling for her. Lucy wants her here."

When my brothers met up with the THON students at a parking lot in State College, Ariana told me how focused my brothers were on getting all of them to CHOP as fast as humanly possible because they were so afraid that Emily would die before they could say goodbye. Jim was also worried about me.

He knows me best of all, as we're only sixteen months apart in age, and he knew that I would stick to my hope for Emily even when the facts were telling any sane person that there was nothing left. He wanted to be at my side for this difficult moment, and he wanted to get there right away. He called our friend Gary, who is a state trooper, to ask him a favor. Please, he asked Gary, tell the troopers stationed on the highway that they were coming through fast on a family medical emergency. He asked that they please not stop them for speeding. Gary said he would take care of it but told them to drive safely to avoid getting into an accident once they hit the interstate.

Becky had never driven this fast before. She later said to me that it was all she could do to keep her eyes on the road at that speed, while Ariana, Kaylee, and Krista were already doing what they could to support Emily. A few weeks earlier, when Emily had been transferred to the PICU, they had started a hashtag on Twitter called #PrayingForEm, and used their connections to THON to encourage people to send Emily love and hope.

The hashtag caught on quickly and was already trending by the time they started on this wild ride to Philadelphia. As Becky was gripping the wheel, Ariana and Kaylee were posting videos describing what was going on with Emily and how they were on their way to represent all the love and good wishes Emily needed to get through this. While they were speeding toward Philadelphia, the numbers of the people following the hashtag started to grow exponentially. By the time they reached CHOP, in a record three and a half hours for a drive that normally takes four, they had thousands more people praying for our little girl.

My mom came out of Emily's room after delivering that message from Lucy. She said she felt filled with love, filled with the grace of the Lord, who she was sure would not turn his gaze away from Emily. She joined me in talking to Dr. Berg.

"You've called your family in, Tom?" Dr. Berg asked me.

"Yes, I have," I said. "Many of them are on their way right now. Emily needs to feel their love so she can pull through this thing."

I could see Dr. Berg struggling to tell me what he truly thought. He is a kind soul, but he didn't want to mislead me or to say anything to encourage my hope in what he saw as a hopeless situation.

"We're the biggest PICU in the country," Dr. Berg began, "and almost every child we put on a ventilator gets off successfully. Unfortunately, I don't believe your daughter will be one of them. Children this sick usually don't get better."

"Please keep trying to help Emily," I said. "I know she is going to get through this."

"You see this line," Dr. Berg said, using his foot to mark off an imaginary line on the floor of the PICU hallway. "I'm telling you this is the line of a body's ability to survive, and Emily is beyond that line. She's walking right along this line and it's like she's walking on the edge of the Grand Canyon. If she gets any worse she'll go over the edge and she'll never come back. Her kidneys are failing, and her lungs are failing. She is not going to be here tomorrow morning."

"I respect your opinion, Dr. Berg, but she's going to make it through this. I'll see you at rounds tomorrow."

I saw that Kari's family had arrived in the waiting room. It was Kristen's birthday, and I know some of the family were holding out hope that Emily would not die that day because it would forever make it a sad observance, not a celebration. I couldn't believe Lindsey was there. She was so obviously pregnant, and it couldn't be comfortable for her to be sitting in those plastic chairs surrounded by people who were in mourning.

I would only allow people in the room one at a time because I agreed with Kari that we didn't want there to be too much going on in that room, as it might drain Emily. I coached people before they entered that when they saw her it would be hard not to fall apart. They had to wait until they felt that they could be strong for Emily, and for Kari. They could see through the glass walls of the PICU that Kari had a scarf around her head to block out the noise of the ventilator and had crawled into the bed next to Emily, carefully twisting her body around the tubes and wires. It was so sad to see this, and at the same time it was such an act of love between mother and daughter.

Kari's mom, Pam, said all the things I thought Emily needed to hear: that she was loved and that she was needed, and that she had to fight with all she had to stay with us because we didn't know how we'd go on without her. That clear-eyed pragmatism that Kari had depended on the day Emily was diagnosed was with Pam at Emily's bedside. She stayed steady and said the right things, no matter how much she was grieving inside.

Robin was next into the room, and I'll never forget the look of shock on his face as he tried to compose himself to speak.

"Miss Em," he said softly. "I know you are going to pull through because we haven't finished our art lessons. I'm still not very good at drawing SpongeBob and I need your help to draw houses right. Miss Em, I need you to keep teaching me."

There was a stir in the hallway when Jim and Greg arrived with Aunt Sally, Becky and Ariana, and the other girls, all still agitated from their high-speed journey. Jim and Greg stood still in the hallway, taking in how Emily looked. Aunt Laurie had arrived a few minutes before. She said to them, "There's no way she survives this. There's no way. Kids cannot survive this."

When Becky saw Emily through the glass to her room, she had to duck out to the bathroom to throw up, she was so upset by what she saw. She had a hard time reconciling the memory from a few days before of the playful way they had washed Becky's car in Kristen's driveway, squirting each other with the hose, with the bloated figure clinging to life on the other side of the glass. Becky knew she had to compose herself because she has no poker face, and she needed to be stronger than that for Emily. This would take a lot of her self-control, and she didn't know how much she had in her. Becky was certain that she and the others had come to be with Emily when she died because, once she saw what Emily looked like, she believed there was no way Emily could pull through.

Aunt Laurie was agitated, more so than I'd seen her, even with all the times we had hit a terrible juncture with Emily. She'd just come off a monthlong rotation at the pediatric intensive care unit at Hershey, which was framing her idea of Emily's chances. She wanted me to have a sober and realistic sense of Emily's odds, not to gin myself up with hope, because the fall from that would hurt so much more.

"I've never seen anyone this sick before, Tom," Aunt Laurie said. "When you have the beginning of multiple organ failure and all of these medicines to support her blood pressure, it's unlikely she'll make it."

"She's still in there," I said. "I know the fight in my girl, and I know she's not giving up. It is not her time."

"They're just keeping her alive on machines," Aunt Laurie said.

Kari started to sob quietly. She knew the truth in what Aunt Laurie was saying. She'd said almost all of that to me. Hearing someone else describe the circumstances Emily faced released some of the sorrow Kari expressed in those tears.

"I've watched six kids die this month, and it was heart wrenching for those families, and for everyone who cared for those children," Aunt Laurie said. "You have a tough decision to make. You don't want to prolong this suffering."

"We've said many times we'll only let her suffer when we know it's leading to a cure," I said. "All this and she's still alive. She's going to be cured."

"Look at the two of you," Aunt Laurie said. "I've never seen you further apart since Emily got sick. Tom, you've always had a way of bringing Kari up, but you can't do that here. You've got to get on the same page here."

"I don't think we can," Kari said.

"You have to sign a Do Not Resuscitate order. I'm saying this for her and for you, too," Aunt Laurie sad. "I've seen so many horrible things happen to children in the PICU. Things that parents should never have to witness. There are a lot of things we in the white coats can do, but should we do them? Not always."

"We have so many people praying for her that I just know, I feel, that the prayers are going to help her get through this," I said.

"My belief in God is not as strong after my husband died in that car accident," Aunt Laurie said. "You do not know why these things happen. Bad things happen and God is not always there. When I saw those six kids die this month, I didn't see God intervening. You have to sign the DNR. If you don't and her heart stops, the PICU team will crack open her chest to try to revive her. You don't want that for Emily. You don't want that to be your last sight of her. You want peace."

"That's not going to happen," I said, although with Aunt Laurie saying all these things it was harder for me to believe the words coming out of my mouth. "Emily's going to make it."

Kari and I went back into Emily's room, she to the armchair and me to the chair next to Emily's bed. It was horrible to see her like that, so swollen that her head was misshapen. Her skin was tight and splotched with purple, and her eyes were taped shut. Kari had taken thousands of photos and videos of Emily in the last two years, documenting every part of the illness. At this moment, when Emily looked so unlike herself, Kari insisted we take no photographs. She did not want to remember Emily this way.

I was lost in my own confusion. I couldn't sign that DNR for Emily because I knew if I did it would feel like I was giving up, like I was signing away her chance for survival. In that way, Aunt Laurie was right about the hope that I clung to so fiercely even at this moment when all the signs said Emily was not going to make it. If she didn't pull through, I'd be a different person on the other side of this. Kari would be, too.

When Robin had left Emily's room, he'd gone to the front desk to ask if they could find someone to give Emily the anointing of the sick. At first they called in a minister, but Robin, being a devoted Catholic, politely told him he needed a priest, so the nurse called another number.

I saw Ariana standing outside Emily's room by herself, and her face was oddly joyful, as though she, of all the other people who were trying to talk straight to me, shared my faith about Emily.

"There's going to be a miracle in that room," she said. "We just have to hold the space for that miracle."

I took her hand and she put her other hand over mine, as if we were praying.

"I'm glad you see it, Ariana," I said. "There's just two of us who do, so we've got to stay strong together."

The monsignor who arrived to minister to Emily performed anointing of the sick, the preparation for being received into the hands of the Lord, to absolve her of her sins so that she could receive the mercy of the church, and viaticum, the Holy Communion that would provide her with spiritual food for the journey to heaven. I watched the priest praying over Emily, and I was buoyed up by his message of hope, not resignation: "God our Father, we have anointed your child Emily with the oil of healing and peace. Caress her, shelter her, and keep her in your tender care. We ask this in the name of Jesus the Lord. Amen."

I know the monsignor could sense my discomfort at his presence invoking Emily's final journey to the Lord. He motioned me out into the hallway to comfort me, too, not just to consecrate Emily's remains into the Lord's care.

"There's been one confirmed miracle at this hospital, and it was a little boy on a ventilator just like your daughter," he said. "He was barely clinging to this world, but he was still here. Two nights in a row, another little boy would appear from the elevator and come to visit the sick boy.

"The sick boy was Chucky McGivern, who was here back in the 1980s. He had smallpox and a fatal kidney disease called Reye's syndrome. His condition was grave. His relatives gave the family religious medals, including one of our local saint, Saint John Neumann, the fourth bishop of Philadelphia. Do you know anything about Saint John Neumann?"

I had to confess that I did not.

"He is a saint of healing," the monsignor said. "There are many miracles connected to him, times when a child was at the edge of death and the family brought the spirit of Saint John Neumann and the child was healed, like this little boy."

The monsignor explained that Chucky's mom, Nancy, said she didn't believe in miracles, except for the chosen, and she didn't feel her family was chosen. Nonetheless, she placed the three medals of the saints on a safety pin, with Saint John Neumann at the center, and pinned them to Chucky's pillow. Her cousin gave her a relic, a piece of cloth from one of Saint John Neumann's robes, which Nancy pinned to the other side of Chucky's pillow.

The next day the doctors told the McGiverns that Chucky had only a 10 percent chance of living; his lungs had collapsed, and his kidneys had stopped working, just like Emily's. The family signed the DNR that I could not make myself sign.

When they returned from signing the DNR, the nurses told the

McGiverns that they'd found a little boy in the room, standing at Chucky's bedside. He was about ten or eleven years old and dressed in a scruffy manner, with a tattered plaid jacket and round glasses, and he had a bowl haircut with bangs.

I was listening intently. A little boy from the elevator? How could this be so?

"The nurses told him he couldn't be there. He needed to go back to his family. When the McGiverns got to Chucky's bedside they noticed that the Saint John Neumann medal Nancy had pinned to his pillow was turned the other way, facing the pillow. That wouldn't be easy to do, I thought. Someone would have to take the pin off the pillow, take two medals off, turn the Saint John Neumann one around, and replace both of them.

Chucky made it through the night, and the next morning, when the doctors were checking him, amazed that he was still alive, the little boy appeared again. The doctors told him he had to leave. He was not family and was not allowed in the room. Chucky's dad, who was sitting in the waiting room, saw a boy who looked just like the one the nurses had described standing at the edge of the waiting room, looking at him. When Chucky's dad stood up and turned to go to speak with the boy, the boy walked into the elevator and the door shut behind him. When the McGiverns got to see Chucky, they saw that the Saint John Neumann medal pinned to his pillow was again turned facing the other way.

Miraculously, Chucky pulled through. The doctors who tended to him said they had never seen anyone this sick get better that fast. A few days later, when Chucky could speak again, he recalled a dream he'd had when he was in a coma. In the dream there was a party for him with many children around his hospital bed, including a little boy whom he described as wearing a plaid jacket, round glasses, and a bowl haircut, just like the mysterious visitor everyone had shooed away from his hospital room.

When Chucky got better, the family took him to visit the church of Saint Peter the Apostle in Philadelphia, the national shrine of Saint John Neumann, to pay their respects and give thanks at the tomb of the saint, who was canonized as the patron saint of sick children in 1977. The church displays images of Saint John Neumann, including a drawing of him as a little boy. Chucky was amazed by this drawing. He told his parents that the boy in the drawing was the same one he saw in his dream.

The story left me speechless. Was it possible that the little boy in the elevator, who had been part of my decisions all this time since I got sick and from the moment Emily had been diagnosed, represented even more than I had attributed to him? I touched my Saint Christopher medal reflexively. The little boy in the elevator meant hope.

"I believe there will be a second miracle confirmed when we are done," I said.

The priest shook my hand and looked me in the eyes in that loving way of deep faith.

"I will be praying for that," he said.

While we were going through this, we didn't realize how quickly the word was spreading about Emily. We had asked for prayers and we got them by the thousands, more than we ever could have imagined. As we sat in her darkened room, the room dominated by the industrial sound of the ventilator that was keeping her alive, I did two things to stay in the neighborhood of hope. Sometimes I would close my eyes and consciously return to the vision I had of the bone marrow transplant hallway where I was teaching Emily to walk. Just her and me, my hand around her shoulders to steady her, as she took one small step and then another with that determined look on her face, and always with just a hint of a smile. She had made it. We had made it, her and me and Kari, and this hellish time in the PICU was all just a memory that set the stage for this incredible victory. Or, after my visit with the priest, I would open my eyes and take my strength from everyone praying for Emily.

The prayers from loved ones and strangers were helping her to survive.

Keep fighting Angel. When you get through this you will be able to face anything. NO mountain will be too big, no river too wide, no hurdle too big. You are an inspiration and you have touched many hearts. We all love you so much and we don't even know you. I know I speak for thousands of people who support you and are waiting to see that you are free from this. Fight angel.
—Cindy Penn-Halse

Hang in there Emily. God wants what is best for you. We are praying for you and your family every day.
—Charlene Coder

Kari didn't have the energy to post when the doctors told us to call in our families to say goodbye, and I didn't share that news on the blog. I wanted the people who were following her progress online to stay in prayer, and not to have any doubts or sorrow. I also knew that we needed their love and support, so I took over posting on the blog to keep our followers engaged. I knew that I needed them as much as Emily did.

Keep drawing your strength from each other and, most importantly, from the Lord Jesus! He is right there beside each one of you at all times, guiding and comforting you, and giving Emily the strength and resolve she needs to fight through each minute and hour of each day. Because of your little girl, so many people—believers and nonbelievers alike—have come together to lift you all up in prayer and even are being drawn closer to the Lord themselves as a result. Fight on Em—you are cared for more than you could ever know!
—Melissa Saupp

We are praying hard in Michigan for Emily's healing and you & Kari's continued strength to support Em through this (awful) experience. I know she can feel your love because we do thru each update you provide to us.
—Cheri Lemaire

I'm praying so hard for Em's strength but also for your (Tom n Kari) peace. I can only imagine the angels surrounding you two and holding you up. Your whole family is being loved and prayed for.
—Angelina Schilt

Keep fighting sweetie. The miracle is happening. You can beat this!!! Kari and Tom hang in there. God is with you and watching over you!!! Your sweet Emily is going to beat this!!!
—Vicki Maines

As I sit here with my 9-year-old girl, every cell in my body is in agony for you...my knees are sore from the time I have spent in prayer for your girl and for you. In the book of Hebrews, the whole of Chapter 11 is a written testament of what God has done through faith...keep the faith, keep fighting Emily and let us do the talking to God...we can do this.

—Joy Swatsworth

We truly believed that, without those prayers, Emily would not have survived that time in the PICU when everyone said she was about to die. The doctors could not explain why she was still alive. We kept telling the doctors it was because of all the support she had and all the people praying for her.

On Wednesday I took Becky and Ariana out to the hospital atrium to speak with them about going home. It was finals week and they were sacrificing a lot to be with Emily, especially Ariana, who had a perfect A average and was certainly risking that by staying with us at CHOP. Some of my family had started on their way home by then and I thought the girls should get back to their lives, too. My brothers were on their way back to Philipsburg. Kari's pregnant sister, Lindsey, also needed to go home, and just in time—just forty-five minutes after she got back her water broke, and she and Pam ended up in another hospital, where she gave birth to a beautiful little girl. Robin and Sharon also headed back home.

Before we left the PICU for our chat in the atrium, Ariana took Robin aside and grabbed his hands to reassure him.

"Don't worry," she said again. "We're going to see a miracle in that room." Robin didn't know what to make of that, but, as a man of strong faith, he wanted to believe, so he chose to do so.

"We can't tell you how important it's been to have you here with us," I said to the girls from THON.

"We don't want to go," Becky said. "We need to be here for Emily."

"And for you and Kari," said Ariana.

"I'll keep you in the loop," I said. "You'll always know what is happening with her. You can't miss finals in your last semester."

"We don't care," Ariana said.

"No, we don't care," said Becky. "There's no place else we want to be."

While we were talking, I got a message from Dr. Grupp, who wanted to talk to me and Kari. He'd been hard to contact in the last day. I would page him, and I know he is responsible about getting back to his patients and their families, but for some reason he didn't get back to me. I didn't spend too much time thinking about this, as I had plenty else to do, tending to Emily, holding on to Kari, and trying to keep my family out of despair. I was trying not to think the worst as I made my way to the PICU and the THON girls came with me to say their goodbyes, still unhappy that I was sending them away.

Dr. Grupp asked Kari and me to step out into the hallway for a chat. He looked tired and I knew he hadn't slept in days while trying to figure out what was going wrong with Emily.

"We've found an anomaly in Emily's blood work," he said. "There's a drug to treat that problem, and with your permission, we'd like to give it a try."

"That's the miracle," said Ariana brightly. "It's all right for us to go home."

Chapter 16

------- ··•·· -------

DR. COWBOY

When I was trying to page Dr. Grupp that night while Emily's life hung in the balance, I thought he was probably sleeping. That's what any sensible person would be doing. Instead, Dr. Grupp was up all night trying to solve the mystery of what was going wrong with Emily. He told me later that he felt a profound sense of responsibility for her. In the first three patients, the older men, they had tried CAR–T cell therapy on, there were some confounding results that might have had something to do with their age. That was what made Emily an ideal candidate for this clinical trial: besides her cancer, all the other parts of her body were healthy, making her a perfect choice to succeed with this treatment. There was no doubt in Dr. Grupp's mind that the things that were going wrong with her were caused by the CAR T cells.

"I had put those cells into her with my own hands, so I felt a profound sense of personal responsibility about what was happening," he said. When he left the hospital to go home that night, he called his wife from his car as he pulled out of the parking garage because he was so fearful for Emily. "I feel like I might have killed that little girl," he'd said.

Late that night, when Emily was stalled at the edge of death, when all the doctors and nurses believed she would not make it through until morning, Dr. Grupp was monitoring her from home on his computer and emailing back and forth with Dr. June, Dr. Bruce Levine, who had modified Emily's T cells, and Dr. David Porter, who supervised the CAR T treatment in the first three adult patients, as well as with Dr. Berg at the PICU, trying to come up with something to save her. The PICU can do amazing things to save a child's life, and the doctors there had done all of those things.

There wasn't much more they could do for Emily. Usually they support low blood pressure with two medications; Emily was on three. She was on the most powerful ventilator they had to support her breathing. They had her on 100 percent oxygen and then added in nitric oxide, which also can support breathing. Many of those IV lines going into her were antibiotics, even though they didn't think her problems were due to infection. Emily was also receiving three blood products: plasma, platelets to control bleeding, and red blood cells because her bone marrow was still not producing them.

As a bone marrow transplant doctor, Dr. Grupp had seen many patients who were very sick, and he knew that most patients who are that sick don't make it. The fact that Emily made it through the night created a sense of urgency for Dr. Grupp and the rest of the scientists working on keeping her alive. As Dr. Grupp later said, "We'd gotten through one night when Emily was not supposed to survive. It's like when somebody climbs Mount Everest. Nobody survives two nights on Everest. We were not going to get her through the next night."

One of the reactions the doctors predicted Emily might have was called cytokine release syndrome, CRS, when large numbers of white blood cells are activated or overproduced, causing inflammation and the production of cytokines, throwing the patient's system out of whack. They call this inflammatory response a cytokine storm, and Emily had some of the symptoms of that: high fever, rapid heart rate, difficulty breathing, and low blood pressure.

In the emails back and forth that night, the doctors didn't know what they should do next. They had given Emily a drug called Enbrel to block some of the inflammation in her immune system, and the steroids, but still she continued to get worse. Her temperature dropped for a little while, but it popped right back up to 104.9.

Part of the scientific infrastructure that Dr. June had built at Penn Medicine was an amazing system of labs to perform detailed analysis and investigation into individuals' tumors, immune systems, and body chemistries so that they could better understand how the CAR–T cell therapy was working. In addition to Dr. Levine, who had developed a groundbreaking method of growing T cells, he had recruited Dr. Michael Kalos, who developed ways to analyze how the infused T cells were expanding in patients, where they were going, how they were functioning, and if they were destroying the tumor cells.

As part of this research, Dr. Kalos had developed a series of biochemical and molecular assays to perform on blood samples they'd collected from patients before the CAR–T cell infusion and every few days after the infusion, so the doctors could monitor any changes. Typically, Dr. Kalos's plan was to run the assessments once a month on all the samples collected so the lab could get a holistic view of what was happening in a patient to identify patterns and trends. Dr. Kalos later told me that doctors generally don't use tests designed for scientific research to make clinical decisions on treating a patient.

But because Emily was so sick and the time was so short and the clinical team could not figure out what was going wrong with Emily using standard clinical tests, Dr. Kalos agreed to run a biochemical test on a week's worth of blood samples, hoping that the tests might reveal something that could help save her life. Usually the full test takes two days to complete, but Dr. Kalos discussed with his lab staff how sick Emily was, and how much scientific research into CAR–T cell therapy depended on trying to save her. The staff agreed to start the tests early in the morning so they could complete the results by the afternoon on the off chance that this information might provide insights that could help save Emily.

But on the day the test was performed, Dr. Kalos was in a bind, a family bind that any father could appreciate. His daughter was a student at a school in Massachusetts, a seven-hour drive from Philadelphia, and he had promised her that he would attend her first lacrosse game that Wednesday afternoon. He knew his being there meant a lot to her, so there was no way he was going to miss it, but he was also very concerned about Emily. The night before, he instructed the lab technicians to send the results to him as soon as they got them. He slipped his iPad, the best device he had to view Emily's results, into his backpack before he left for Massachusetts that morning.

As he was standing on the sidelines cheering his daughter, he heard the ping that announced an email from the lab. Dr. Kalos walked away from the game and opened up his iPad to assess the results.

"Holy moly," he remembers saying when he saw them. The results showed that Emily's CAR T cells were really revved up and strong. They had chewed through the steroids and continued replicating at a robust rate. The other thing that jumped out for Dr. Kalos was that Emily's blood had a very high level of interleukin 6 (IL-6) protein, a protein involved in inflammation, usually associated with other immune cells and, at the time, not associated with CAR–T cell therapy.

Dr. Kalos immediately forwarded the lab results and his interpretation to Drs. Grupp, June, and David Teachey, another specialist in leukemia who has his office near Dr. Grupp. In the minutes before they all jumped on a conference call, the doctors were frantically trying to chase down what this elevated level of the IL-6 protein meant to Emily's immune system, searching scientific studies, and trying to find other doctors who had addressed this issue.

On a call Wednesday afternoon, Dr. June sounded very excited by the elevated IL-6 protein because his daughter, who is just a few years older than Emily, has juvenile rheumatoid arthritis, which also produces elevated levels of IL-6. In following his daughter's care, Dr. June had been tracking treatments for that.

"Steve, my daughter has juvenile rheumatoid arthritis," he said. "It's an IL-6 immunity event, just like this. There's a drug for this. Do you think the pharmacy has any tocilizumab?"

"How is this going to work to help Emily?" Dr. Grupp wanted to know. "No one has ever used this drug on a cancer patient before. And IL-6 isn't even made by T cells."

"It's not a widely used drug," Dr. June said. "But it does work on this."

In a situation like Emily's, where the patient is critically ill and the doctors are not sure what is going on, they had to try something they wouldn't try under normal circumstances. Taking a chance was better than doing nothing. Still, a number of things had to work out for Dr. Grupp to give the drug to Emily. First, he had to find out if the pharmacy had it. If they did not, it was likely that they couldn't get it in time to save her. The distributor usually gets the drug to the hospital within twenty-four to forty-eight hours from when a doctor orders it, but they didn't have that long. Dr. Grupp called the pharmacy, and he found out they had two vials.

Then he had to convince the pharmacist it was ethical and logical to give a leukemia patient a drug that is prescribed only for juvenile rheumatoid arthritis. Research hospital pharmacies are cautious about off-label uses for drugs. Dr. Grupp and the pharmacist discussed how he was going to use the drug with Emily. Thankfully, there was already a pediatric dose approved in the package insert. Dr. Grupp advised that he was going to follow those dosage instructions and the pharmacist signed off on allowing him to prescribe the drug. The next hurdle was the PICU staff.

Dr. Grupp decided to make his case in person. With the vials of tocilizumab in hand, Dr. Grupp walked into the PICU to talk to Dr. Berg about their idea. He knew if anyone along the way said no, they wouldn't have anything left to try. He knew everyone he spoke with wanted the best for Emily, so what was the best? Did the drug pose another risk? Everyone wants what is safe, and *safe* and *best* sometimes don't overlap. This was one of those moments. Basically, he decided, what he was trying to do was to convince other medical professionals that he and Dr. June weren't nuts.

One of the reasons the barriers were falling, and falling quickly, was because it did not look like Emily would make it another twelve hours. A decision had to be made quickly. Dr. Berg and Dr. Grupp had a spirited conversation, with all of those values at play. Dr. Berg agreed that if Dr. Grupp had found something that gave Emily a chance to pull through, even if it was unconventional and perhaps risky, they had to give it a try. He signed off on the tocilizumab, with a grin of respect.

"You guys are cowboys—you know that, don't you?" Dr. Berg said.

The top rung on the permission tree was me and Kari. Dr. Grupp came to us with the wind at his back. I didn't know what was putting the spring in his step, but I sensed his fresh energy.

"We're grasping at straws, but we have an idea," Dr. Grupp started off.

By 8:00 p.m. the tocilizumab was in Emily.

—··●··—

Chapter 17

#WEBELIEVE

The doctors just rounded with us. Emily's right lung is re-inflated and showing up on the X-ray. The doctor used the term "amazing" when describing her lungs from yesterday to today. He said you can't get better until you stop getting worse. He said Emily is no longer getting worse and is starting toward getting better. He also said this is the reason why you never give up on a child's chance of coming back.

—Kari's journal

April 26, 2012

That evening when Emily received the tocilizumab, all we could do was pray that it worked, but we were not prepared for how quickly that happened. A few hours after it was administered, her fever disappeared. She'd suffered with a fever somewhere between 103 and 106 since Sunday, and suddenly it was gone. Although she was improving, she had a long distance to go before she was considered to be better.

The PICU doctors were concerned because, after days of lethal low blood pressure, a few hours after she received tocilizumab, her blood pressure started to climb into a dangerously high range. As a bone marrow transplant doctor, one of the things Dr. Grupp worried the most about with his patients was the dangerous combination of high blood pressure and low platelets, which is what Emily suddenly had. If left untreated, these two things combined can cause significant bleeding in the head. Dr. Grupp called the PICU to discuss with them immediately taking Emily off the three medicines that were supporting her blood pressure. Generally, doctors take a patient off a medication slowly because it's safer, but in Emily's unusual case, faster was safer. The doctors didn't have as much experience in trying to take a patient off that blood-pressure-boosting medication so fast, as it usually takes a long time for a patient's blood pressure to regulate. They didn't know how long it would take for the drugs to work their way out of Emily's system.

By dawn, less than twelve hours after the first dose of tocilizumab, Emily was off two of the three blood pressure medications. When Dr. Grupp came in the next morning, I could see he was as tired as we were, but I also saw relief. He had watched Emily's breathtakingly quick steps to recovery on his laptop from home. Her miraculous progress was a huge contrast from the twelve hours that had preceded that, when he was out of ideas, out of hope, and casting about for any solution.

"I have seen patients get better, and I have been grateful when they get better," Dr. Grupp said. "I have made decisions that have helped patients get better, but nothing like this. As I watched Emily's numbers change last night, watched her heal in real time, I thought, oh my God. How is this possible?"

Where had I heard that question before? From the story of Chucky McGivern and his visit by the boy in the elevator.

Kari and I had watched the concerned actions by the nurses and the doctors as they cared for Emily that night. We were now pretty good at reading the machines, but we didn't have the skills to understand the whole picture. We were not prepared for Dr. Grupp's optimism.

The other good news from Dr. Grupp was that the CAR T cells appeared to be holding their own in the battle against the steroids. We had agonized for hours about whether to give Emily steroids to help her lungs because Dr. Topjian had told us about the research that showed steroids sometimes killed off T cells. Emily's CAR T cells never paused in their fight. They just kept on multiplying. Amazing.

"You're saying she's better, Dr. Grupp?" I asked.

"She's still critically ill, but she's improving," he said. "We have taken multiple steps back from the cliff, but the cliff is still there. What we need now is for nothing else unexpected to happen."

----------··●··----------

The cliff was still there, and we were still on its edge. And while Kari and I were excited about the first real progress Emily had made in the week since she got that last infusion of CAR T cells, our support network outside Emily's PICU room was still praying as hard as they could, not knowing that, along with the medicine, the prayers were starting to work. I wanted them to know not to give up that hope because she still needed it.

I asked Kari if I could write on the blog and she turned the computer over to me. I could see how exhausted she was and that she was not ready to describe what was going on with Emily, not just yet. After Dr. Grupp's visit, I wanted to communicate with the thousands of people who—I could tell from the messages they left us—were getting up in the middle of the night to check on what was happening with Emily, whose first thoughts in the morning were to wonder if she had made it through the night.

Emily fought through the night and we are seeing some small steps forward. They were at the maximum settings on the ventilator to support her breathing yesterday. They suctioned her lungs and removed some mucus and overnight they turned down the oxygen from 100% to 46% and she held her own...her kidneys aren't where they need to be, but they should improve. Em's blood pressure and heart rate are OK today and the war continues. Kari and I are pulling strength from the fight in Emily because it is brutal for us to see her like this.

—Tom (writing in Kari's journal)

April 26, 2012

I flashed back to that evening before, when Ariana agreed with me that, against the odds, a miracle would happen and Emily would pull through. I wasn't so sure Becky was on the same page as Ariana and me. Becky was in agreement in one way, though: she believed in raising as many prayers and positive thoughts as she could, and Kari and I agreed with her about that.

"We're going to go home and we're going to raise some hell," Becky had said as they told us goodbye.

"We're going to rally so many prayers and so many thoughts," Ariana said. "Let's do this. We'll get all the people who are on the Facebook page to come out and pray for Emily."

They later told me that they didn't talk much during the ride back to Penn State. They were so overwhelmed by the days they had spent crouched on the floor, sleeping in chairs, subsisting on Subway sandwiches and energy gum, up all night praying, that they didn't have anything left to say. They had all been there for Emily, and for us, spending all their energy holding on to the hope that Emily would make it through the night, and she did.

After they dropped the other girls off, Becky and Ariana sat in the driveway holding each other and sobbing, letting it all go. Ariana can't recall if they sat there for a few minutes or a few hours, but by the time they had finished sobbing, they were determined to come up with a way to support Emily from Penn State.

The hashtag #PrayingForEm they had made before they left for CHOP, the one where they had been posting live updates of their own, now had thousands of followers. It had started strong with the other members of their PRSSA club sharing the message with their families and their friends at Penn State, at THON, and beyond. While they were with us at the hospital, as the precariousness of Emily's situation increased, the audience grew and grew. It leaped even further with my message of hope on the day they left, the day when Emily started to turn around, when I posted, "I believe I am witnessing a miracle."

"I believe" was what I truly felt, even though Emily's fight was far from over. The followers of the Prayers for Emily Whitehead Facebook page quickly transformed that into the #WeBelieve hashtag that, while the girls were making their way back to Penn State, had started to trend regionally on Twitter and Facebook. People started posting photos of themselves wearing Emily's favorite color purple and holding up signs that said "#WeBelieve" and "#PrayingForEm."

When they got back, Becky and Ariana remembered that great birthday party we'd had for Emily the summer before, when she had to have three parties: one for the family, one for her kindergarten friends, and one for her college friends. With the help of those great publicists at PRSSA, they encouraged Emily's college friends to gather in the student center at Penn State—the HUB—to sing happy birthday to Emily. They coordinated this idea even though Emily's birthday was a week away, because they believed that with more hope, more energy, Emily would make it to the age of seven.

That night, before they went their separate ways to get some sleep, they posted the invitation on Facebook, hoping that somebody, even if it was only a few people, would be willing to take the time away from their finals to sing to Emily. They told everyone that they intended to record it and post it, and also that they would send it to us to play in Emily's room on her seventh birthday. The day after they arrived home, one of their friends, Nick Hope, made a happy birthday banner for Emily. Becky and Ariana unrolled that banner in front of the student bookstore, encouraging passersby to write happy birthday messages on it for Emily.

That afternoon, Becky and Ariana gathered up the banner from the bookstore and made their way to the HUB, and their jaws dropped. They had expected they'd see some people from THON and more from PRSSA, plus a few others, but the whole place was full. The HUB is a big open space with a long, wide stairway leading up from the main floor, where Ariana and Becky planned to unfurl the banner. A balcony where students gather to eat and to study wraps around the open space. The whole floor of the HUB was jammed with students and there were hundreds more crammed onto the balcony, ready to sing to Emily.

The two girls stood at the top of the stairs in awe.

"This is going to do it," Ariana said to Becky. "With so many people here, how could this positive energy not get to Emily in Philadelphia? All this love from all these people who support her."

"You have to get real about this," Becky said. "She's not going to make it."

"She's absolutely going to make it!" Ariana shouted back.

"The priest came and gave her last rites!" Becky shouted.

"And she's still here! And he said there could be a miracle!"

"You and Tom, you have to get off of your cloud and back to the real world," Becky said.

So there they were, two girls whom everyone knew as best friends, who had only come together because of Emily, standing in front of hundreds of people at their student center screaming at each other at the tops of their lungs.

Off at the edge of the crowd someone started to sing "Happy Birthday," and the strength of that song grew as more and more people started to join. Becky and Ariana looked up from their argument and grabbed their cell phones to film the moment. Even if it was still in doubt whether Emily would make it, these students at the HUB were not going to let that stop them from wishing and praying for Emily.

———— ··●·· ————

At around the same time Becky and Ariana were coordinating the idea for the birthday sing-along in the HUB, my brothers were arriving back in Philipsburg. Jim was so exhausted that all he wanted to do was go home and get some sleep. He hadn't seen his family in days, and he knew he was scheduled to work the next day. He just wanted to slip into bed and try not to think about what was happening with his niece. Both he and Greg were pretty sure it wouldn't be long before they were back on the road to Philadelphia to support me as I watched Emily die. Maybe there would be a moment—and it wouldn't be too long—when I would have to decide, as Jim had told me to do, that I had to let Emily go. Unthinkable as that was, against everything they knew about me, they knew that they would be there to support me if it came to that. Their mood was the same as the one that had colored the car ride home for Becky and Ariana.

Just before they got to Philipsburg, Jim got a call from Big Jim telling him he couldn't go home, not just yet. Some people were organizing a vigil in support of Emily at Cold Stream Park and Big Jim wanted someone from the family to provide an update on Emily to whoever showed up.

Jim does not enjoy public speaking and, anyway, this was about the last thing in the world he wanted to do that evening, but he said yes. When he and Greg rounded the driveway into the park, their jaws dropped. There were hundreds of people along the shores and more crammed into the amphitheater at the back of the area around the dam. There were policemen and firemen, as well as large church groups, Girl Scout and Boy Scout troops, kids from surrounding schools, guys from our union and our job, and people from our family church of Saints Peter and Paul.

Jim knew his voice would never project loudly enough for all these hundreds of people to hear, so he asked Gary if he could borrow the loudspeaker from the patrol car. Gary handed him the microphone and he stood with his feet in the floor of the patrol car so all the people who were there for Emily could see him.

He started off slowly, talking about how Emily was fighting, but it was a big battle, and the battle was a tough one for a little girl to win. He talked about her in the intensive care unit and how the monsignor had come to perform the anointing of the sick.

Back in Philadelphia, I don't know what came over me at that moment, but something whispered to me that I needed to call Jim, if only to make sure that they all got home safe. I had no idea that he was in the middle of a speech.

He was speaking when he saw my name on his cell phone. And he interrupted what he was saying.

"Hey! It's Tom calling!" he said, and he remembers the murmur that went up from the crowd. I started describing what was happening in

Emily's room at that moment, and he repeated everything I said into his ear right into the microphone.

"Emily's fever is down," he said. "They're trying to take her off these blood pressure medications really fast because her blood pressure is back to normal....And Tom says the last X-ray shows that her lungs are starting to clear up."

Someone from deep in the crowd yelled out, "WE BELIEVE!"

And the call came up from all over Cold Stream Park to answer that back. People from all over shouting, "WE BELIEVE!"

That evening, when Becky and Ariana organized that huge sing-along and all those people gathered at Cold Stream Park to pray together for Emily, had not been an easy time between me and Kari. I was buoyed up by Emily's amazing improvement and by all the positive energy that I had sensed coming from hundreds of miles away. We may have seemed like fools when we were rushing from one thing to the next in search of something to save Emily, but whatever we'd done, it was working. I had gone on the blog to tell the world that Emily was pretty much cancer free. Kari deleted the post, and we got into a huge argument.

"You cannot be out there declaring 'She's cured!'" Kari said. "All Dr. Grupp said was that he was 'cautiously optimistic.' He didn't say she was better."

"Let's focus on the good stuff, Kari," I shot back. "Something's working. We just don't know what it is yet. Her white cells are up, way up. That's the T cells working."

"You're always Mr. Positivity, and sometimes it makes me crazy," she told me. "I just cannot get my hopes up. Usually when her white count is up that means the cancer is growing again. I need to see her labs to know what's going on."

It was good that just then Dr. Grupp came into the room to settle our argument. In some ways, it was still the science-versus-faith contest that had been going on between us since Emily got sick.

"I've got some interesting news about Emily's blood work," he said.

"Interesting" news was usually not good news for us, I thought.

"The B cells are disappearing from Emily's blood," he said. "There is only one reason why this would be happening."

"The CAR T cells are working! They are killing the cancer cells!" I exclaimed.

"It appears that the steroids didn't harm them after all," Dr. Grupp said. "In fact, she has more CAR T cells in her bloodstream than any of the men who were treated with this therapy had at this point."

"They're working!" I said.

"Don't get too excited," Dr. Grupp cautioned. "We see the T cells but we're not sure what they are doing yet. We're going to run more tests tomorrow."

"I'm pretty excited, Dr. Grupp," I said. "Emily's still fighting."

"This is a marathon, Tom," Dr. Grupp said. "And I'd say Emily is about on mile four of this race. Her numbers are getting stronger and she's not giving up, but there's still a long way to go."

Yesterday Emily was on mile 3 of her marathon for her critical care and today she's on mile 4, so she's making progress. She's starting to wake up from sedation, so they have to give her "rescues" which means they give her an extra dose of sedation meds to make sure she's still asleep. She's had a couple of these episodes this morning, which is unnerving for us because we do not want her to be aware of what's going on. She's able to maintain good blood pressure on her own now. They also lowered the settings on her ventilator and will test for a certain type of pneumonia kids with low immune systems get. Her kidney function is moving toward normal again and her liver function is also better. This is good news, but we don't know what the cancer in her bone marrow is doing.

—Kari

The moral of a story we were told this morning was that it is not the size or the stature of a person you judge them by but judge them by the shadow that they cast. We were told of a man who, because of that story, has started signing his email "IN EMILY'S SHADOW" before his name. WE BELIEVE!

—Tom

(writing in Kari's Journal)

April 28, 2012

For the next three days, Emily was better in some measures and worse in others. She'd breathe a bit better and they'd reduce the amount of pressure on the ventilator to encourage her to breathe more on her own. Then her oxygen levels would start to plummet, and they'd have to increase the pressure on the ventilator and increase the sedation so she could tolerate that. If she started to surface from unconsciousness, she would realize there was a breathing tube in her throat and that, along with the noise of the ventilator, and all the tubes and lines coming into her body, would make her blood pressure rise, so they'd give her even more sedation. By Sunday the swelling in her body had decreased dramatically. Emily started to look like Emily again, and Kari noticed that her eyelashes and her hair were starting to grow back.

Occasionally, she would open her eyes, and the moment she did we would be up on our feet trying to reassure her that everything was okay. Kari was ever at the ready with the stuffed Lucy dog we had nearby, as we knew that always cheered Emily.

"Everything is okay, Emily," Kari said to her. "Just stay calm."

"You don't know how much support you have, Emily," I said. "Becky and Ariana were here and many other students from THON. There are thousands of people praying for you. And everyone is really excited about your birthday."

"Your birthday is only a few days from now," Kari said.

"Yes, and it's going to be great!" I added.

We didn't know if what we said was reaching her. The minute the nurses saw that we were talking to her and she seemed to be responding, they gave her stronger sedation and she was back in that dark silence again.

In the days before her birthday they switched the oscillating ventilator to one that was less powerful and less noisy because X-rays showed her lungs starting to clear up more. Emily looked and seemed more comfortable, but I was not. I had a flare-up of my Crohn's disease that was so severe I had to be hospitalized, too. This was two kinds of agony for me, not just the physical pain but my sorrow that I was not there for Kari and Emily and my fear that I would not be there for her birthday. I was ecstatic when they discharged me the day before Emily's birthday.

On Emily's seventh birthday everyone in our family and all her fans throughout the country and the world were grateful that she was still alive to celebrate. She was doing great on the less-powerful ventilator. In fact, she was doing so well that they started to wean her off the paralytic medicine so that she would gradually wake up. Kari and I were afraid she was awake but too paralyzed by the medicines to be able to open her eyes. Several hours a day we would stand by her bed talking to let her hear that she was loved and that we were certain she would wake up soon, and we were even more adamant about this on her birthday.

"Emily," I remember saying, "it's your birthday and it's a beautiful day outside."

"It is, honey," Kari said. "The sun is shining and it's going to be summer soon. We know how much you love the summer."

"Yes, summertime," I said. "Uncle Greg started heating up the pool so it will be warm and ready for you when you get out of here. We'll go swimming every day. All you have to do is wake up."

Emily started to blink her eyes open.

"I'll go tell the nurses!" Kari said. We'd promised the nursing staff that, if we saw her waking up, we'd let them know right away. There was a good chance Emily would panic when she woke up enough to feel the breathing tube and her instinct would be to pull it out. We couldn't have that.

We told the nurses, who came rushing in to stand around her bed and sing "Happy Birthday" to her. While they were singing, Kari and I each took one of Emily's hands. As we reached the end of the song, Emily squeezed our hands! I felt a sense of relief even with that one little flutter of her lashes. Just a week earlier she'd told me she didn't have the strength to fight anymore, and here she was, responding. Shortly after our celebration, the nurses had to increase her sedation again, so she'd keep that breathing tube in, and she went back into dreamland. The biggest birthday gift the doctors gave us was saying it was possible that she could be off all ventilator support within the next two or three days.

Over the next few days, they stopped the antibiotics and slowly decreased the other medications. We counted down as the nurses removed each of those seventeen IV pumps one by one. Kari and I would talk to her, reading her stories and reminding her of things from home, trying to get her to breathe some on her own.

"Lammy is here, waiting for you to wake up so you can cuddle. Did you know that? She's right here and I'm holding her. And Lucy is waiting for you at home, so you have to get better and see her. Everyone loves you so much, Emily. There are people all over the world praying for you, and the doctors here are taking such amazing care of you. I know you're going to pull through this," I'd say, or it would be Kari's turn and she'd say something similar.

Soon Emily was awake enough to shake her head yes and no when we asked her questions and she could point to letters to spell out things she felt, like telling us, "I miss Lucy."

We were anxious even though Emily was doing better. She was scheduled for a bone marrow aspiration later that week that would show if she had any cancer cells left in her blood or if the CAR T cells had killed the cancer cells as they were designed to do.

Kari didn't want to get her hopes up because there had been so many times when she had, only to have them dashed by bad news. I reminded her that this time was different. We had thousands of people praying for Emily and supporting her. We had spent the last week sorting through the hundreds of cards from strangers whose lives had been touched by Emily's fight to live. I thought there had to be a reason the steroids never killed her T cells when the doctors had been so certain that they would. I felt there had to be a reason why she'd made it through the night when the doctors were sure that she would not. There was no medical explanation, so it had to be something bigger. I was willing to hope—but then, that's my job!

Chapter 18

———— ··●·· ————

WITNESSING A MIRACLE

On May 5, the doctors and nurses were holding back tears as they removed the breathing tube from Emily and turned off the ventilator. They had thought they would take the tube out only after she died. None of them anticipated that she would be so well two weeks from the moment when she hovered on the brink of death that they would be able to remove it. I had posted on the Facebook page, "We believe," and many of the comments we received on that post echoed my sentiment, but it was most gratifying to see it in the tears on the faces of the people who had worked so hard to keep Emily alive.

Emily was weak from being in a medically induced coma for two weeks and couldn't sit up or hold her head up on her own for very long. I wasn't complaining at all, though. The fact that she was alive was a miracle, delivered to us directly by the incredible doctors and staff at CHOP, the prayers and support of our amazing family, the little boy in the elevator, and by the thousands of people all around the world. When I posted "I believe," I was believing in all of that, of course, but also in the remarkable strength and tenacity of our little girl. Everyone was certain she would not make it through the night when Dr. Berg drew the line with his foot on the PICU floor and said she had already crossed over it. We had called in our families to say goodbye, and she was still here. We'd gotten through the hardest part, but we had yet to see if the CAR T cells had killed the cancer cells.

> Emily is getting a little stronger each day. She's able to support herself a little more when she sits up. Doctors completely stopped one of the sedation meds she's been on, but she had withdrawal symptoms all day, throwing up and just not feeling well. She was able to talk better today—her voice was a little stronger. Tomorrow (when they will examine her bone marrow for cancer) is a very, very big day. It's hard to get my hopes up after we've had our hopes up so many times before only to receive bad news. However I feel like there has to be a reason she made it through the night when the doctors said she wouldn't. There has to be a reason that the steroids never killed the T cells when the doctors were so certain that they would. We've heard from the doctors that there isn't any medical explanation for some of the things that happened. We Believe!
>
> —Kari's journal
> May 9, 2012

Besides Emily's bone marrow aspiration, the doctors had also ordered a CT scan because a few weeks earlier, they'd noticed a nodule on one of her kidneys and they wanted to make sure it hadn't grown. After Emily's bone marrow aspiration, I went with her into the CT scan room so I could be with her as she got her scan. Kari was in a waiting room across the hall. My eyes were on Emily, but my mind was worrying about the bone marrow results, which the doctors promised they would get to us as soon as they knew.

The scan takes about twenty minutes. Emily was starting to emerge from the tube when my phone rang. I saw it was Dr. Grupp!

"Hello?" I said, my heart pounding.

"Tom, this is Steve Grupp," he said. "I'm in New Orleans at a conference, but I wanted to be the one to tell you. It worked. Her bone marrow shows no sign of disease. There is no leukemia. Emily is cancer free!"

From the waiting room, Kari watched me walk into the hall and I could see her face stricken with worry.

"What's wrong?" she asked, slowly walking toward me.

"The T cells worked!" I said.

"It worked?" she gasped.

"She's cancer free," I said in a broken voice as I started crying.

She ran to me and I hugged her tightly in my arms. It had happened. Our prayers were answered. We had finally received the news we had been waiting for. The whispers had guided us to this miracle. As I held Kari, both of us sobbing in the hospital hallway, as we had so many times in the past two years, I felt a huge weight lifted, as if the elephant that had been sitting on me had just stood up. From the beginning I'd told Emily she would get better, she'd believed me, and it had finally happened. Our family made it.

I called my parents and Kari called hers to start the family grapevines going. By the time Emily was out of the procedure and back in her hospital room, our phones were ringing, but we didn't answer. We knew we had to post an update to Emily's supporters. There was so much to say, but for now a brief post was all we needed.

No cancer cells! T cells worked!!!!

—Kari's journal

May 10, 2012

In the days after Kari posted that Emily was cancer free, we experienced how much the world had been praying for our girl. Hundreds of messages of celebration came shortly after we posted the message that Emily was cancer free.

Wow, I'm sitting here just speechless, wondering what to say that can sum up everything in one word. The only thing I can come up with is BELIEVE.
—Christina Daniko

YAAY! This brought great tears to my eyes and my heart overwhelmed with so much joy and happiness!! God has really blessed Emily, she is a true miracle! What a trooper Em...We love you!
—Keena Lorrine Wilson

I just burst into tears....Thank you Lord for answering so many prayers....We have witnessed a miracle, albeit via Facebook. Congratulations to the entire family....Emily you are such an inspiration, am sure your journey will help so many other people. Keep fighting girl!
—Ellie Helen Fulkerson

Praise God!
—Kathy Coursen

Amen!

—Lori Orndorff

AMEN!!!!! WE BELIEVE!!!

—Bernie Strong

The doctors continued to test Emily's bone marrow via several tests, trying as hard as they could to find the tiniest sign that there was still cancer there, but they could not find one cancer cell.

We had asked the world for prayers and it had come through stronger than anyone could have imagined. As the word spread through the hospital that Emily was cancer free, parents and relatives of other children at CHOP came to place their hands on the glass front of Emily's room because they wanted to feel the miracle. The word spread from there out through the blog, and people started coming to CHOP trying to get up to the PICU to visit Emily for the same reason: they wanted to get close to this miracle. Several times complete strangers evaded security to get up to our floor, and we had to speak to the staff about stronger measures to protect Emily. I felt such sympathy for them, as they were at the place Kari and I had been, clinging to hope, but this was for Emily's health and for her safety.

The next hurdle was to help Emily regain her strength.

Three days after they pronounced her cancer free, the nurse came into Emily's room with a broad smile on her face.

"This is a big day for you!" she said. "You're getting out of the PICU."

Emily perked up at this news. The PICU nurses had promised to throw her a big birthday party as soon as she was transferred to the oncology floor.

"Dr. Grupp is on service this week in the bone marrow transplant hallway," she said. "We're transferring Emily there so he can watch over her care."

"The bone marrow transplant hallway!" I grinned and looked at Kari.

"Yes," said the nurse. "Emily's still very weak, and once you get settled in there, I want you to work on getting her to walk."

"I've looked forward to helping her get back on her feet," I said.

"Start off slow," the nurse said. "Her muscles haven't been used for weeks. She's not going to want to do it and it will be very painful for her at first. You'll need to use tough love."

"Love is the toughest thing I know."

"The aides will be here soon to help you move," she said, and left.

I looked up and Kari was smiling at me, her head cocked in that charming way where her hair is lush at the side. I could see she had joy in her eyes again.

"I'm never going to doubt your whispers again," she said.

———— ··●·· ————

A few hours later, we unpacked our heaps of decorations and stuffed animals and boxes of books in the very same room on the bone marrow transplant hallway Dr. Bunin had showed me the first day we visited CHOP. I was itching to get Emily up on her feet and walking, and Kari was watching my restlessness with a sideways grin. Emily was asleep and sleep was important, so her antsy dad was not allowed to shake her awake.

Finally, Emily was awake, but she wanted to eat and then Kari and she had to read a book or two. It was like they were torturing me, letting this happen in its own sweet time when this was the most important thing in the world at that moment as far as I was concerned.

"Emily, the nurses say the only way you're going to get back on your feet is to get back on your feet," I said. "C'mon, let's take a loop in the hallway."

"No, Daddy," she said. "It hurts to walk. It hurts when I stretch my legs."

"I'll help you. I'll be right at your side there, holding you up just a little so it doesn't hurt so bad," I said. I swung her legs out of the hospital bed and scooted her forward at the edge to put a little pressure on the tips of her toes.

"Ouch!" she cried.

"Let's go really slow, now," I said. I eased her down off the bed as slowly as I could, and Kari brought around her walker. Emily was on her tippy toes, wary of letting her heels hit the floor because her muscles were so tight. I could hear a little whimper from Emily as she tiptoed lightly, taking such tender steps that if it wasn't for the sound of the IV pole I was dragging behind, the bags of fluids sloshing against the side, we'd have made no sound at all.

Making it out of the room was the answer to my prayers. Emily, however tentatively, was taking steps on her own. I was the proud dad, the man with his heart about to burst. During the darkest moments of Emily's illness, every time the news was bad, as with the relapse, and every time the cancer came back stronger than before, and that night when they all said she wouldn't make it, I had clung to this very image. It was a dream come true to me, an accomplishment, a deeply desired victory—for Emily most of all, but also for me and Kari. And here it was a reality, hesitant, tentative, but one that seemed to have been supported by the whole wide world.

Chapter 19

HOMECOMING

As we prepared to bring Emily home, people all over the hospital were calling it a miracle. So many of the nurses and staff had been there next to us when no one thought Emily would make it through the night, and they were there to celebrate with us when she did. It was more than that, though. This was bigger than just the survival of one little girl. If Emily hadn't survived, research into this way of killing cancer would have stopped. It might not have been funded again for many years. She had carried so much hope, and so many people's lives, on her little shoulders, and she almost didn't make it.

As we were piling all the cards and books onto a cart we borrowed from the hospital, Dr. Grupp came into the room to say goodbye, and to thank us. We were the ones who wanted to thank him, so the feeling in the room was all joyful. This crazy idea of using the body's immune system to treat cancer had worked, and it opened up so many possibilities for future treatment. Dr. Grupp told us that the director of the National Institutes of Health (NIH) heard about Emily's recovery and all he could say was "Wow!" Emily's victory meant that there would be more research to improve this treatment and other scientists finding ways to apply this personalized method in other types of cancers.

There was a tender feeling among us because of the pride we all had in Emily. When Emily had nearly died, we all felt it, and so did people around the world who were following the blog. This was a profound bond we shared with Dr. Grupp, the medical staff, our friends and family, and with many people we would never meet.

"You know, Tom and Kari, I don't know how you made all those decisions for her treatment, but they ended up being the right ones," Dr. Grupp said.

"Yeah, a lot of that time it wasn't easy to decide," I said.

"We tried our best," Kari added. "I studied the scientific literature, but most of the time we questioned every decision we made."

"All those times we went against the doctors' recommendations," I recalled. "Like when we turned down the chemo at Hershey and came here."

"And then we turned down the clinical trial here and went right back to Hershey again," Kari said.

"And all that time we spent waiting for the bone marrow donor," I said, remembering the agony we felt during those weeks when we didn't know what to do.

"The reason I ask how you made those decisions is this," Dr. Grupp said. "If you had agreed to the ICE chemo at Hershey, or the temsirolimus at CHOP, Emily wouldn't have been eligible for this clinical trial. She never would have gotten the CAR T cells."

"Those were difficult decisions," I said.

"You've given me a few gray hairs," Dr. Grupp joked.

I reached over to hold Kari's hand to acknowledge all we had gone through together and how, against all the odds, we ended up getting it right. One of many miracles in this room.

"Dr. Grupp, did you have faith that Emily would make it? Did you believe?" I asked.

"Optimism is not faith," Dr. Grupp said. "You can hope for the best. From my perspective, if you start allowing that to drive your decisions, then you are not looking to the downside as a possibility. If you hope the patient gets better, that's awesome. Hope is a very powerful tool. It is what keeps me going and keeps the families going as long as it is not unrealistic. But belief steps beyond what we know, and that is what you have to be careful of from a physician's point of view. I view it as part of my job not to let belief substitute for judgment. I believe my role is to be ruthlessly objective. Given the fact that I am a human being and I care a lot for these patients and I desperately want them to get better, I have to be as objective as I can."

"So you don't think what happened to Emily was a miracle? How she survived that night was just good luck until science could save her?" I asked.

"Oh no, I'll say miracle, but I might mean something different when I say it," Dr. Grupp said. "When she pulled through that night, it seems miraculous to me. In the medical world we talk about error reduction and we describe how all holes in the Swiss cheese have to line up for an error to get through. This was the opposite. The Swiss cheese holes had to line up so that Emily could survive, and if you shifted any of those just a millimeter, it doesn't happen. I'm fine with calling that a miracle."

"We think it's one," I said.

"We do," Kari affirmed.

"And we want to do whatever we can to help spread the word about this treatment so other parents know it's available to save their children fighting cancer," I said. "If you ever need a family to talk about this treatment or for us to share our experience, you should call us."

"Thank you," he said. "We'll stay in touch. And now you get to take your little girl home, cancer free."

As I loaded up the car, Kari checked our Facebook page, where she saw that it seemed the whole world was celebrating Emily coming home, especially our friends and family around Philipsburg. In the days when we were waiting to bring Emily home, people in Philipsburg kept posting that they were planning to line the streets to welcome us back. As we set off from Philadelphia, we didn't think that would happen. There was a storm predicted to come through Philipsburg right when we were going to be pulling into town. This was not just a spring shower, either, but a real deluge. We didn't expect anyone would come out during a thunderstorm.

We settled into the car, Emily in the back in her booster seat and Kari at my side. For the first time in months, our normal life was there to reach out and take back again.

As we pulled onto the turnpike, I remembered the crazy drives we took: all of the ambulance rides, the time I almost got a gun drawn on me by the police, all the times we were stuck in traffic with Emily sick in the backseat, me groggy because I hadn't slept in days or doubled over in pain from my Crohn's. All of that was behind us now, with Philadelphia getting farther and farther away in the rearview mirror.

I kept glancing back at Emily, awed by the strength and tenacity in my little girl. I remembered the boy in the elevator years before, when I was at Johns Hopkins, and how calm he was, and the same little boy that the monsignor described to us at CHOP. That was never Emily. She was feisty, full of life, no matter what the disease threw at her. From the moment I held Emily in my arms as a baby, I heard a whisper that she was going to do something great. Here she was only seven, and she had already done something that had changed the world. She had changed the way we treat cancer.

We were still a family, and we were stronger because of all that we had been through together. I had always loved Kari, but now I knew her deeply and, also, she understood me. Our marriage was stronger and even that felt like a miracle. Our love and respect for each other deepened.

And I had a stronger sense of faith, too. Maybe it wasn't the same as anyone else's, but it was all mine and it was very strong. I could say to anyone that I had proof that miracles happened and that my whispers were real. To everyone who doubted my whispers, I could explain with confidence that, if you don't lose hope, things you can only dream about can come true. I had always felt my faith most strongly when I was in nature, but now I knew how to recognize it in unexpected places as well. I saw the brotherly faith in the lodge in our hunting camp. All of us bunked in an open room above a big, dark porch, talking late into the night and sharing the family folklore. I recognized it, too, when Jim and I flew loose-limbed over the hills on our dirt bikes, jumping high in the air, unconcerned about a fall. I know faith in my marriage. And I felt it coming from all the people I'd never meet who prayed and hoped for Emily. Although we didn't know them, we always felt the steady stream of love and support coming from Emily's supporters all over the world. Together we made this miracle.

My cousin Jodie kept texting me as we drove, asking where we were on the journey back home. She wanted to know the exact time we departed CHOP. Every stop we made along the way—when we needed a bathroom break or when I stopped for gas—I felt I needed to check in with Jodie, although I wasn't completely sure why she was so concerned.

About forty-five minutes from Philipsburg, we hit that torrential downpour that the weather service had warned about, rain so dense it was hard to drive, and pulled over at a convenience store to get a drink and, of course, to update Jodie on our progress. I voice-texted her when we got off the freeway and made the turn home, and Kari texted her mom, who was waiting for us at our house along with many other family members and friends.

Jodie texted, telling me to stop at the bowling alley because she had a surprise waiting there for Emily. There were two state trooper cars and three fire trucks in the parking lot. We'd been amazed by the support from the firefighters, who did a boot drive for Emily. They'd stood at intersections holding out their big rubber boots, asking people to toss in money for Emily. That one day they raised $4,500! The state troopers said they were there to guide us home and make sure we were not stopped by traffic as we drove through town. Suddenly, our one-family car was part of a parade of fire trucks and police cars.

"You know people want to see Emily," Kari said. "You might want to put her in the front seat so that if there is anyone on the street when we drive through, they can wave to her.

"It's pouring out here." I said. "I don't think there'll be anybody on the street."

"I think you should do it anyway."

Kari was right. Emily should be in front for her homecoming, even if there were just a few people hardy enough to stand on the streets to welcome her. It took us a minute to switch everything around so Emily's booster seat was on the passenger side, but Emily was not impatient. She was enjoying the prospect of a parade to welcome her home. The only thing she really wanted, she told me, was to see Lucy.

The fire truck at the front of our little parade hit the siren as we started down the long road to the center of town. Emily stared out the window excited by how the town had turned out to welcome her.

"Daddy, look!" she said. "All the trees are covered in purple ribbons!"

Kari had her phone up, snapping pictures as we drove. Clusters of families, dozens of them, huddled under umbrellas and all wearing purple T-shirts they'd bought at fund-raisers. Hundreds of people stood at the roadside in the rain holding up purple "WE BELIEVE" signs.

At the center of town, there were many more, people hanging off the sides of trucks or standing up in the backs of pickups, faces of schoolkids poked out the windows of family cars and vans with voices yelling: "Welcome home, Emily!" "We love you, Emily!" "We believe!" Later we found out that they had let school out early so that all the kids who had contributed so much love and support, and so much birthday money, could see Emily return. Almost every car we saw had a purple "WE BELIEVE" sticker in the rear window.

Through the tears in my eyes, I looked back at Kari and saw the tears in hers. It dawned on me that Emily was not just our little girl; she was everyone's.

We had another stop to make before we got home. Jodie told us to pull over at my grandmother's house, which is right on the route. There we saw a photographer from our local paper, *The Centre Daily Times*, my grandma, mom, and Big Jim holding Lucy. I looked at Emily, so pale and with dark circles under her eyes and the feeding tube still inserted into her nose. It looked as though she was too weak to hold up her hand. Then she saw Lucy and the sparkle returned. I rolled down her window and Lucy leapt out of Big Jim's arms and right into Emily's lap.

"Emily, don't let Lucy lick your face!" Kari said, ever watchful of germs, but there was no interrupting this moment. Emily was suddenly filled with energy, most of it provided by Lucy.

As we continued home, there were people lining the streets along the country road that leads up to our house, at the turn up the hill leading to our street, and down the block, all the way until we pulled into our driveway, where the local news station reporters and their cameras stood there to greet us.

As we helped Emily out of the car, Lucy was running back and forth, her tail wagging. Emily picked up Lucy and gave her another kiss. There would be no interviews that day, at least not for Emily. Inside, the whole family was waiting to welcome her.

At last Emily had come home.

WHAT'S HAPPENED
SINCE EMILY CAME HOME

Last year, our family flew to Miami, as we now do most years, for a world stem cell conference that brings together doctors, scientists, CEOs, and hedge fund managers from around the world interested in finding out the latest advances in the CAR–T cell therapy that saved Emily. After we tell our story to the crowd, the conference organizers usher us onto a large yacht, one that can hold hundreds of people, which sails down the Miami River in the moonlight. At the banquet, we were seated next to a CEO who had heard my talk, and he beamed with excitement as he swept his hand around the large crowd. "Without Emily Whitehead, none of this is possible," he said.

I am proud of my girl in so many ways. First off, I'm proud of her for just being her, the same strong and spirited girl she was before she got sick, the same girl who never gave up and the one who changed the way doctors treat cancer. If Emily hadn't survived, this treatment approach that already has saved hundreds of lives would have been delayed by years, perhaps decades. If a healthy young girl like Emily was not able to get better, scientists might have given up this research, at least for a while, if the treatment put patients at risk. But the fact that she survived, and continues to thrive, gave doctors the freedom to treat more patients with CAR–T cell therapy, and to begin researching the use of CAR T cells on other forms of cancer.

When we got home that June afternoon in 2012, none of this was certain. Yes, Emily appeared to be cancer free, but there were anxious moments at every checkup when we wondered if the CAR T cells were still in there, still fighting off Emily's leukemia. Every time we took her to the doctor, we confirmed that she was still cancer free. In December of that year, Dr. Grupp presented the results of the first few patients treated with CAR–T cell therapy, Emily among them, at a meeting of the American Society of Hematology. This was what led to her being featured on the front page of the *New York Times*, where they accurately depicted our daily joy in Emily in the first paragraph of the story, describing her somersaulting around the house and taking tumbles that "made her parents wince."

The reaction to this article was huge! More than 550 articles were published in the U.S. about Emily's treatment in the two weeks after the *Times* article. Hundreds more were published around the world. From that moment on, our family was called upon to speak to large groups and small ones. We told the story of Emily's miraculous cure with CAR–T cell therapy and spread the word about this lifesaving treatment. Many times when we spoke, the scientists who work in the laboratories, the front line for this research, would echo what the head of the National Institutes of Health (NIH) told us. When NIH director Dr. Francis Collins invited us to lunch, he told us he kept a picture of Emily on his desk as a constant reminder of why he came to work every day. Other scientists and researchers told us that, too.

Something about the magical nature of the cure, and of Emily's story, kept drawing attention her way. General Electric sponsored a series of short films, called *Focus/Forward*, that features new ideas in science. They commissioned one on CAR–T cell therapy and Emily, called *Fire with Fire*, by Oscar-winning director Ross Kauffman. It has been viewed more than 20 million times.

Emily's cure was a big boost as well for Dr. June, who had relied on grants and philanthropic contributions to finance his research. With the publicity generated by Emily's and others' survival, big pharmaceutical companies came courting, wanting to license CAR–T cell therapy for worldwide distribution. He chose Novartis to be his partner. The company contributed $20 million to Dr. June's research, financing a huge new facility for him affiliated with the University of Pennsylvania called the Center for Advanced Cellular Therapies (CACT). It has 24,000 square feet of lab space, 6,400 square feet of clean room space, and 100 scientists who can tailor treatment for 400 patients a year. When the center opened in 2016, Dr. Levine, the scientist who grew Emily's cells, joked that Yankee Stadium was the house that Ruth built, but Emily built CACT.

The desire to celebrate this novel approach to treating cancer kept our whole family on the go, speaking at conferences and to researchers, scientists, and pharmaceutical and biotech companies around the world to inspire their workforces. Everyone was eager for this story, including VICE, which did a program on new kinds of precision cancer treatments, including Emily and CAR–T cell therapy, in 2015 called *VICE Special Report: Killing Cancer*. And we got to know and become friends with documentary filmmaker Ken Burns when he featured Emily's story as the last segment in his PBS documentary *Cancer: The Emperor of All Maladies*.

Around this time, we were thinking that we could use all the attention Emily's story was getting to start a foundation in her name. We wanted to bring news of the treatment to a broader audience of parents who were at the exact place we had been: given a hopeless diagnosis and told to move their child to hospice. Between ten and twenty times a month, parents from around the country (and, later, from around the world) called me to ask if their child's situation was like Emily's, or to ask for a referral to a doctor or a hospital that could offer them the same therapy. I always take those calls. As I remembered from those afternoons with the other pediatric cancer parents in the outpatient oncology clinic, and from that grandmother at the family lounge in those first days at Hershey, only we knew what each other was going through. We needed to be kind to everyone we met.

The other goal of the foundation was to fund research for less-toxic treatments for pediatric cancer. We knew a lot of cancer foundations were raising money off the bright news of Emily's survival, but some of them didn't donate to pediatric cancer research. We talked about setting up the Emily Whitehead Foundation, but we weren't sure when would be the right moment to launch. I was the one who was gun shy, but Kari had better sense than me. She was listening to *her* whispers. I'm the one who is always forwarding positive memes and sayings, so much so that it can get to be a little annoying. While I was hemming and hawing, Kari sent me a meme! It said, "What some people see as obstacles others see as opportunities." That was all it took for me to decide. We launched the next week, and a few days later Emily was invited to the White House, a great sign that our timing was perfect.

When I was teaching Emily to walk again on the bone marrow transplant hallway, I used to tell her that what she had done to fight cancer was so big, so earthshaking, that one day she would meet the president. You can imagine the eye roll I got from her when I said that! But sure enough, when President Barack Obama announced his Precision

Medicine Initiative with strong bipartisan support, he invited Emily to come to the White House. We could see why her story fit perfectly into this event. It was so promising that it was the kind of approach that gave people hope that we actually could cure cancer. Also, I was bursting with pride for another reason. Any dad can tell his daughter she'll meet the president one day, but my prediction came true!

2017 was Emily's five-year anniversary of being cancer-free, and at her check-up with Dr. Grupp he pronounced her cured. Just a few months after that, the FDA approved CAR–T cell therapy for use nationwide. Since then it has been approved in several other countries. In our little corner of Pennsylvania, we all felt like we had a piece of that victory, no one more than Emily.

What we had wanted for Emily was a normal, small-town life, but fate did not agree with that modest goal. She's had something much different in the last eight years, meeting celebrities and world-famous leaders, appearing on television, and speaking before thousands of people. Our families are still the same, still supportive, loving, squabbling, and knit even closer together than before because of what we all went through when Emily got sick. Becky and Ariana are still Emily's dear friends, so much so that Emily was a bridesmaid at Becky's wedding. Every time we go to New York City (which is now one of my favorite cities!), the three of them sneak off together with plans of their own, and it makes me so proud that that relationship continues. Emily can look to those two young women as role models for what Kari and I envision for Emily.

Our foundation is five years old now and has raised more than $1.6 million. In 2017 we held our first Believe Ball, named after the #WeBelieve hashtag that rocketed around the country when Emily was close to death. At the ball, we honor the doctors and researchers who developed CAR–T cell therapy and who care for pediatric cancer patients.

We also honor the patients and their families. We're holding another Believe Ball in fall 2021.

Every time I'm asked to tell Emily's story, I do it with pride for how we got through it and pride in the amazing young woman Emily is today. I might tell that story fifty or more times in a year with all the speaking I do, and every time I do, I break down in tears. It is as if it was happening right now, the feeling of it is so powerful to me. I'll never forget what happened, and if it chokes me up to talk about it, so be it. It's too important not to talk about it if it could save the life of another child.

———··•··———

To learn more about the Emily Whitehead Foundation please visit www .EmilyWhiteheadFoundation.org.

AFTERWORD

by Emily

———··◉··———

Since I got well, my family has traveled the world to help promote the treatment that saved my life. My story has inspired many and made them feel close to us, even if they have not met us. Everywhere we go, somebody recognizes me. From strangers on a plane yelling. "Oh my god! Emily's on this flight!" to people telling me how they found out about my story. It never gets old. I love to hear how my story has inspired others. Many people are taken aback by how much I have grown. Eight years later, people are still baffled that I'm not a seven-year-old girl anymore. It still baffles me that people of all ages admire me, and say that I am their hero, for a part of my life that I do not remember a lot about. My parents gave up everything for me, and being in the hospital for so long made us close. I am extremely grateful for my life, and the memories I would not have if I had not made it out of the hospital. Currently, I am a typical teenager that has just a few more life experiences than the kids in my grade.

One of the things that was most important to me during my years in the hospital was Lucy. I hazily remember the day she visited me in the hospital, but I know that she made me want to recover and come home so that I could see her again. Before I became sick, I had begged my parents for a dog. Being the strong-willed child I was, I was determined. That begging came to a halt when I was diagnosed, but it left a lasting impression on my parents. They had seen how quickly the kids' moods would change as soon as they saw one of the therapy dogs come onto the floor at Hershey. That inspired them to get me Lucy. I don't remember the day she was given to me, but I remember how close we became in the following years. Unfortunately, Lucy passed away in June of 2019. She had heart and lung issues that led us to having to put her down. My dad even drove her to Philadelphia to see a special veterinarian to see if anyone could fix her. Lucy and I had a special bond that left quite the impression on my family. She grew up with me and helped me through a very rough time in my family's life. In my heart, this book is dedicated to Lucy.

My dad understood how much I needed Lucy and was always trying to find ways to have her visit me at Hershey and CHOP. Besides being the person that made me laugh every day, he also enjoyed tricking me.

Whenever I had enough energy, my dad would walk me down to the playroom at Hershey, dragging my IV poles for me so I could feel somewhat free. I called him my IV boy because I always refused to drag the poles myself. The playroom had glass walls on the back, overlooking the woods and buildings surrounding the medical center. There were crafts, games, and even a Nintendo Wii lined against the front wall. These are regular activities for any sick child in the hospital. Although these activities were fun, directly outside of the glass walls entering the playroom stood a neon-green-and-blue air hockey table. While the other kids played inside the playroom, I would play intense games of air hockey with my dad outside of the playroom.

Any chance my dad could get, he tricked me. His tricks ranged from saying Lucy was behind me, to trying to convince me that my mom needed me. During our first competitive days at the hospital, I would always turn around. He would chuckle and score the puck into my goal. As I grew more accustomed to my stay at the hospital, I became more focused on every game of air hockey we played. It wasn't long before I caught on to his tricks and outwitted him myself. Today, my dad and I play air hockey games on any air hockey table we can find and, of course, still use the same tricks.

Besides playing air hockey games with my dad, I needed some entertainment in my hospital room when I was put in isolation for having a low immune system. Typically, books and stuffed animals kept me occupied in those long hours trapped in that small space. On one of my mom's posts, she explained my obsession with stuffed animals and reading. Little did we know what was to come. A few days after that post, I received hundreds of books and stuffed animals from our supporters on Facebook and CaringBridge. My mom and I read those books back and forth to each other throughout the rest of my treatment. The support we received was amazing and inspired me to keep fighting.

After I relapsed, I became a different kid. I was bald and I had a better medical education than many adults. I could even explain the medications I needed and why I needed them to my nurses and could change out my own syringes. I received steroids that made me shout so noisily that the entire oncology floor could have heard me threaten to fire the group of nurses who came in to see me. That girl that was in the hospital did not feel like me.

One day, I felt as if I needed a change. I decided to tell everyone to call me Emma. For the next two years, that was my name. After I came home from the hospital after CAR–T cell therapy, I started to feel like myself again. I knew that I could go back to being Emily. I never understood why I did this until I became older. Now I recognize that I needed some way to separate the real me from who I was in the hospital. When

I changed my name back to Emily, I left my past behind me in the hospital. Emma was that sick girl in the hospital, with no hair, who played air hockey at the playroom. She fought relentlessly until the very end and overcame any obstacle that faced her. As soon as I became Emily, I started to share my story with the world, and that is who I am today.

Being the first child to receive CAR–T cell therapy, I've been able to experience things the majority of people don't get to experience in their entire life. I've traveled to Switzerland, France, Germany, Canada, Norway, and Sweden. With all the trips we've taken to promote CAR–T cell therapy, I've discovered that I really enjoy traveling, especially overseas. Out of all of the places I've traveled to, Switzerland really had an impact on me. My first trip to Switzerland was in June of 2015, three years after I came home from the hospital. When I boarded the plane to endure the eight-hour flight, I did not know what was to come.

When we were about to land, I decided to pull up the window shade for the first time since we had taken off. The glare of the morning light lit up the cabin as my eyes adjusted to the new landscape. I remember the mountains with their snow-peaked tops and the blanket of green trees wrapping around them, so tall that their peaks touched the clouds. I had never seen anything like that until I pulled up that window shade. It seemed like an entirely different world from the rolling hills of Pennsylvania. I've been to Switzerland twice and got to explore the Swiss Alps, see cows wearing bells, and eat some of the best food I've ever had.

Besides traveling around the world, I have met some pretty neat people. While I was in the hospital, my dad always told me he knew that I was going to meet the president someday. My mom would tell him to stop telling me that, but he seemed determined, like he somehow saw it happening. In 2015, my dad received a call from an unknown number while he was working in his bucket truck. The caller explained that

President Obama mentioned me in his Precision Medicine Initiative, his campaign to promote cures like mine that individually tailor the genetics, environment, and lives of people who get sick. He wanted me to be there for his next speech! I think my dad almost dropped his phone out of his hand. A few weeks later, I was able to meet President Obama. He even signed my school excuse slip so the teachers would not doubt the reason I was absent. It was an amazing experience that I'll never forget.

A year later, Sean Parker, a Silicon Valley investor, was inspired by the death of a close friend to start a cancer immunotherapy foundation, the Parker Institute for Cancer Immunotherapy. He invited my family and me to come to a fund-raiser at his home in Beverly Hills. There, I met people like Katy Perry, Bradley Cooper, and Lady Gaga. Usually, my dad would tell my entire story and let people meet and talk to me after, but that night I had my first small speaking part. I was nervous to speak in front of such a large crowd, especially one filled with celebrities, but I was determined to do just as well as my dad did during his speeches. After saying a few words onstage and eating a good meal, Lady Gaga came out onto the stage and began singing "La Vie en Rose," the same song she later sang in *A Star Is Born*. While she was singing, my dad pointed down at me and she pulled me up onstage and sang to me in front of the crowd. It felt like a dream. I watched her twirl her scarf around onstage and dance next to the trumpet player as the crowd swayed and cheered her on.

Another gala that we attended was for *TIME* magazine in 2018. Dr. June was in the top 100 most influential people of the year, and I got to write his tribute. I explained in a few short sentences that he was my hero and had saved my family. At the gala, I was able to meet Millie Bobby Brown and Shawn Mendes and I shook hands with J.Lo. The night seemed like a dream, and it was a remarkable experience.

When I was in the hospital, I found a love for art. I would paint and do crafts to decorate the dull walls of my hospital room, and I never stopped. I still love art, but I've also found a passion for film. Throughout all of our interviews and short films, I've always been interested in what happens behind the scenes. My love for film became stronger when Steven Spielberg's team reached out and wanted me to be in his Dream-Works short film about innovative ideas and inventions in 2019. He ended up including my one-through-six-year "cancer free" photos that my mom takes every year on the anniversary of the day the doctors declared me free of the disease.

The film premiered in the Comcast building in Philadelphia on a screen in a large spherical theater specially built just for it. While I was there, I was able to meet Mr. Spielberg and explain my new passion for film. A few months later, he let me spend a day on set with him so I could see what happened behind the scenes. I got to see the actors in action for the remake of *West Side Story*. The sets were located in a large building that was filled with people. We toured multiple sets that were condensed next to each other, and there was even an entire store that was filled with objects inspired by actual goods from the 1960s. One thing that really interested me was how many people are required to make one movie. There were at least a couple hundred people just in the building working on it, compared to the usual crew of five that came when someone interviewed us at home. It was astounding to see Mr. Spielberg in his working environment. While on set, Mr. Spielberg actually sent a video of him and me together to President Obama on his phone. That was definitely something I will remember for the rest of my life.

When we saw the impact my story had on other people, my family wanted to make a bigger difference. My parents and I created the Emily Whitehead Foundation, which raises money for pediatric cancer patients. We've raised over a million dollars and hope to raise more to help families find less-toxic treatments with immunotherapy and get out of the hospital for good. More than 1,000 patients have been treated, and would have likely passed away without CAR–T cell therapy and the money to fund the research. We raise money by hosting a Believe Ball that gathers all of the CAR–T cell therapy patients together for a night to give them an experience they won't forget. At our first Believe Ball, I brought a group of friends that made it especially memorable for me. Seeing all of the CAR–T cell therapy families gathered in one place inspired me to continue to raise awareness for pediatric cancer and get my story out there even more.

Currently, I go for doctors' appointments every year and was entered into the survivorship clinic at CHOP. My dad does most of the traveling to conferences, but any overseas trips or visits to California, I'm in on. I go to school with the same classmates I started with in kindergarten. I was able to keep up with my work by reading with my mom and the tutoring I received from the incredible teachers at the hospital and from my local school. I keep up with my schooling even now with my travels. I hang out with my friends and I look forward every day to coming home and seeing our new chihuahua, Luna.

A couple of months after Lucy passed away, we longed to have a dog in our quiet house again. We found several adorable chihuahua puppies online and decided to make a bond with a dog again. I kept the *L* names and went with Luna, and I am glad I chose that. Lucy's loving spirit is in Luna's, and Luna is just as spoiled as Lucy was. Luna always wants to know where I am and gets just as excited as Lucy did when we get home from traveling. Unlike Lucy, Luna is a ball of energy that always keeps us on our toes. Despite her bursts of energy, she still has a love for napping. To represent them both I wear a necklace with a star that represents Lucy and a moon to represent Luna.

Being the first pediatric CAR–T cell patient means so much to me. When I was younger, I could not understand why I was receiving so much attention, but as I grew older, I began to understand how important it is for other families and their kids to hear about my story and make it more accessible around the world. I am so thankful that I was able to be the first pediatric patient for the treatment and help so many other kids make memories that they never would have been able to make. The experiences I've had and memories I've made are all because of my family, our supporters, and my doctors. I want to continue to spread my story around the world and inspire other young adults to make a difference and stand up for what they believe in. Together we can write a better story for kids and young adults around the world.

———— ··●·· ————

In the words of my dad, remember to smile every day. You never know when something could change in an instant.

ACKNOWLEDGMENTS

In the retelling of our journey, we did our best to be accurate based on our memories of the events, our journal entries, and interviews. A few things have been changed for privacy or narrative purposes. Thank you to those who took the time to be interviewed and provide input for our book!

Thank you to our incredible CAR T team at CHOP and Penn Medicine: Dr. Stephan Grupp, Dr. Carl June, Dr. Bruce Levine, Dr. Michael Kalos, and everyone who worked on the CAR–T cell therapy. Because of you, we get to see Emily grow up!

To our CHOP doctors, nurses, and staff in the PICU and oncology unit, including Dr. Alexis Topjian, Dr. Robert Berg, Dr. Susan Rheingold, and so many others, thank you for the incredible care you provided for Emily.

To the doctors, nurses, and staff at Hershey Medical Center—without your amazing care, Emily would not have made it to CAR–T cell therapy.

Thank you to Dr. Jim Powell for the care you've shown in treating Emily and the guidance you provided. Also, thank you to the Mount Nittany Medical Center ER staff and nurses Kayla and Marsha.

And thank you to the child life specialists, social workers, and music and art therapists (and pet therapy dogs!) who work so hard to make things easier for families trying to navigate a new reality in the hospital.

Although only a few people from Penn State THON and PRSSA are mentioned in the book, there are many who are important to us. We are grateful for the fun and laughter you brought to Emily during the most difficult time of her life. We can't imagine not having the support of our THON family!

To WME and Hachette Book Group, thank you for helping us make our book a reality. To Danelle, thank you for working with us and bringing our story to life. To Ken Burns, thank you for your guidance and belief in our story. And to Lynn Ann, thank you for your friendship and advice throughout the past eight years.

To our friends, community, and supporters all over the world—we never could have imagined the response we received when we asked for prayers and positive thoughts. Thank you for every prayer and fund-raiser and for every comment on our CaringBridge and Facebook posts. These helped tremendously during our darkest days.

To the CAR–T cell therapy and pediatric cancer families, you inspire us every day to keep sharing our story and raise awareness for less toxic pediatric cancer treatments.

Thank you to our incredible family!

We Believe!

ABOUT THE AUTHORS

The Whitehead Family

Tom, Kari, and Emily Whitehead are cofounders of the Emily Whitehead Foundation, which raises funds and awareness for pediatric cancer immunotherapy research. The foundation was created in honor of Emily, who was diagnosed at age five with an aggressive form of leukemia that failed to respond to chemotherapy. As a last hope, Emily was enrolled in a clinical trial and became the first child in the world to receive the pioneering cancer treatment called CAR–T cell therapy. The therapy worked, and Emily remains cancer free. Emily's story has been featured in Ken Burns's PBS documentary *Cancer: The Emperor of All Maladies*, HBO's *VICE Special Report: Killing Cancer*, the *New York Times*, the *Washington Post*, *Parents* magazine, *CBS Evening News*, *NBC Nightly News*, *ABC World News Tonight*, Fox News, CNN, and the Stand Up to Cancer telethon. The Whitehead family travels worldwide as keynote speakers to inspire others and advocate for research funding to develop less-toxic childhood cancer treatments. When they aren't traveling, Tom works as a journeyman lineman for Penelec of First Energy, and Kari is a registered dietitian and research project manager. Emily attends high school and plans to become an artist or filmmaker. The Whiteheads live in Central Pennsylvania with their chihuahua named Luna.

Danelle Morton

Journalist and author Danelle Morton has collaborated on sixteen books including four *New York Times* bestsellers.